OPTIMIZE YOUR HEALTH WITH THERAPEUTIC PEPTIDES

EXTEND YOUR LIFE BY BECOMING MORE MUSCULAR, LEANER, SMARTER, INJURY-FREE AND YOUNGER

BY JAY CAMPBELL

FOREWORD

I first met Jay after reading his 2018 hormonal optimization masterpiece *The Testosterone Optimization Therapy Bible*. I interviewed him for the first time on my podcast in early 2019, and I remember the conversation well. At the time, Jay and I had a disagreement about the safety of the drug metformin. But as a lifelong student of human optimization, I like to get as many informed perspectives as I possibly can, so I wanted to sit down with him to see if there was something that I'd missed...

Our conversation was nothing short of spectacular. Speaking with Jay fundamentally changed my mind on metformin. Through his insane attention to detail, he was able to point out nuances in the research I'd previously been unaware of. We ended up talking for over two hours that day, covering a wide range of topics, and I was absolutely blown away by his depth of knowledge on optimizing the human body - **especially when it came to peptides**.

Since then, Jay has been on my podcast two more times, discussing all things health optimization, and I consider him to be both a collaborator and a good friend. Jay truly stands out as a leading voice in the health optimization community, and it's my pleasure to introduce this latest book on using therapeutic peptides.

His newest book *Optimize Your Health with Therapeutic Peptides* is an absolute masterpiece.

As someone who both personally uses and educates the public on peptides, I truly believe these compounds represent the future of medicine. Peptides have long been kind of a secret weapon of functional medicine physicians and biohackers, yet they remain mostly ignored or unknown by mainstream medicine and the general public.

Jay's book just might change that.

What truly makes his work so special is how *accessible* it is. Because peptides still exist outside of the awareness of most physicians, YOU, as the end user, are unfortunately left to navigate this world alone.

Now, Jay's book is the solution. Jay has done what so few experts in this space have been able to do. He's taken all the complex science of therapeutic peptides and presented it in a way completely understandable to the average person.

Simply put, Jay's book will tell you everything you desire to know about using therapeutic peptides within the context of health and longevity.

Jay has stripped away all the fluff and left you with exactly what is necessary - a clear, concise guide and seamless action plan for harnessing the power of these incredible compounds to heal your body, dramatically improve your health and (for many) completely transform your life.

Ben Greenfield

Health consultant, speaker and New York Times best-selling author, BenGreenfieldLife.com

AUTHOR'S INTRODUCTION

People are slowly starting to wake up.

They're realizing the "sick care" model of allopathic medicine has failed them.

This awakening has only accelerated over the last two and a half years thanks to government and Big Pharma's utter incompetence, if not outright malfeasance.

Allopathic medicine is a sinking ship.

It's a model fundamentally predicated on treating the symptoms of illness and dis-EASE while ignoring their root causes.

The sad fact is that visiting most doctors today with an illness or injury is like taking your car to a mechanic because the engines on fire… only to have them slap some duct tape on it while sending you on your way.

Peptides are the exact opposite of the slap-dash, too-late, "medicate the symptoms with drugs" model of health.

As of this very moment, peptides are lighting the health and biohacking communities on fire due to their ability to fundamentally solve the root causes of illness and disease.

With over 20 years in the optimized health industry and having used therapeutic peptides for more than 14 years, I AM convinced peptides are truly the now and future of regenerative medicine.

For over ten years, the entire Jay Campbell brand has been dedicated to helping men and women maximize their health without introducing harmful substances into their bodies.

Physical avatar bodies have already been ravaged by the modern American diet and mostly sedentary lifestyles.

Peptides can and are changing the future of health, medicine, and healing forever.

Not only do they get to the root cause of the issue, but they also offer the ability to treat illness from a fundamentally regenerative approach.

They work with your body to encourage and rapidly accelerate the natural process of healing.

You may not realize it, but right now you have a unique opportunity...

Because so many of these trends come and go "usually with more sizzle than steak", you may be skeptical.

You may be wondering how simple compounds made

from mere amino acids can *truly* deliver on the hype they've been generating.

I've been in this game for a long time, and I've seen some remarkable things, but the stuff I've seen with peptides can only be described as a miracle.

I've seen lifelong, nagging injuries plaguing people for years that turn around in a matter of weeks.

I've seen people accelerate their fat loss in ways I didn't think were possible.

I've seen, and personally experienced, profound improvements in cognition, focus, and energy levels.

When used in conjunction with a healthy and optimized lifestyle, peptides are the real deal.

As you'll soon find out, the interest and buzz they've been generating over the last few years is absolutely justified.

The ways in which these compounds can be applied to the human body are nearly endless. This gloriously concise book is designed to get you familiar with them.

You'll learn exactly what peptides are and why they're so incredibly versatile.

You'll also learn what NOT to do: the mistakes that you

absolutely must avoid getting the most out of them.

Finally, you'll get an overview of the most common kinds of peptides available on the market today, and which ones are best suited to your health issue.

If you're ready to start harnessing the power of these incredible compounds while ultimately taking control of your personal health, let's dive in.

TABLE OF CONTENTS

Chapter 3: The Best Peptides For Fat Loss ... 57

Chapter 4: The Best Peptides for Longevity . 89

TESTIMONIALS FOR JAY'S WORK

Tailor Made was the 4th fastest growing company in healthcare almost entirely due to our expertise and introduction of peptides into the clinical market.

When we first launched, Jay was the first person to interview us about the work we were doing.

Jay realized the impact of, and potential of, these peptides even then and has continued to be THE leading expert in this field.

I highly recommend reading his insights if you are considering peptide optimization.

Ryan Smith
Former Founder of Tailor Made
Compounding and Founder of TruDiagnostic

I have known Jay for 10 years now (how it's been that long is crazy to me).

Jay is a genius-level intellect who also happens to be a hardcore bro, who is deeply spiritual. He has educated himself into one of the foremost experts on testosterone, hormonal health, health enhancement and life extension.

He has also published multiple books and courses on the topics of therapeutic testosterone, peptides, fasting and life optimization– each of which is in a league of its own.

Jay is also more knowledgeable and a better teacher than 99% of personal trainers. He has designed multiple supplements that work better than anything else in their class.

His talent stack is ridiculous. Jay is a real Polymath. Said simply, "If Jay says something 'works', it DEFINITELY WORKS. Jay Campbell DOES NOT BULLSHIT!"

Alexander Cortes (AJAX)
#1 OG of Fitness Twitter

I am almost 62 years old and have worn many hats in the fitness industry over the last 35+ years.

I am always in pursuit of the most up to date cutting edge research and science regarding human optimization.

I have learned from many experts in the optimization space, but Jay stands alone and miles ahead of the rest at the top!

Welcome.. you have purchased the right book….get ready to learn!

Jeff Seidman
61-Year-Old Certified epigenetic and nutrigenomic coach,

trainer to celebrities, supermodels and professional athletes and featured on television, radio and in hundreds of fitness magazines

My brother,

You are a light in the darkness of this world. I really appreciate you and your wife.

You were the impetus for getting me on testosterone in 2016 which has improved my quality of life immensely.

I have several your books, your peptide course, and I use your hair regrowth products on my hair to allow me to look great at 53.

I wish the world had listened to you about the v-shots.

I am looking to bring my gf down to Mexico soon for stem cells. All of that is because of your integrity, honesty, and hard work. You really are improving people's lives.

Kevin Ryan, SSG, US Army, Ret.

Jay,

Just wanted to say thank you again. Everything is really falling in line with my life and my family's life. Physically, we haven't been better.

Mentally, man, you really helped me through your podcast. It allowed me to be open to meditation and positive thoughts. Complete game and life change, over the past year.

Please don't stop spreading the message of health, fitness, and positivity, brother.

Nathan

Hey Jay,

I've been listening to your podcast for several years now, learned a bunch when it came to health and training, and a ton more when it comes to the more spiritual topics.

Just wanted to show you some love and gratitude.

Keep up the good work.

I appreciate you and so do so many others.

Adam

NOTE FROM THE AUTHOR

Thank you so much for purchasing this book and any of my previous books.

It is my great honor to serve you.

I hope you find this book enjoyable and enlightening for your journey on the path to regenerative healing.

If you are reading this book expecting me to validate and justify my conclusions with published or peer reviewed research, you've come to the wrong place.

If you are an "evidence-based scientism-ist," seeking validation and scientific "research" to substantiate my claims, you just lost your investment.

You've been fooled into thinking studies are foolproof, credible and valid when they are NOTHING OF THE SORT.

Studies today are almost worthless and certainly cannot be taken at face value from anyone.

Most of their designs have been manipulated to achieve a specific result, and the great majority of studies cannot be successfully replicated.

They're often written in complex language, making them difficult to interpret. One must learn how to "study the study" and "follow the money."

There are many who live and die by the "infallible" scientific method, and yet they fail to see its inherent flaws and biases.

To make matters worse, the statistical methods used in most studies are such that *"if measurement errors were to be taken into account in every study in the social sciences, nothing would ever get published"*[1].

The linked article covers social sciences specifically, but the issue is present across all fields.

A brief Google search will even show you the dirty underbelly of modern research.

From false AI-generated studies readily accepted by major publishers, to intentionally hiding known faked results so every study based on those fake results doesn't get rejected, it's almost shocking what people can get away with.

Dr. Anthony Jay's paradigm altering book **Estrogeneration**[2] conclusively proves most studies are fraudulent.

For massive amounts of scientific research and clinical validation, read my first 3 books.

---

[1] http://pepbk.co/ReplicationCrisis
[2] http://pepbk.co/Estrogeneration

This book (and any future book) is written for explicit instruction on how to use therapeutic peptides to become fully optimized in all aspects of one's health in the most effective and efficient way possible.

MEDICAL DISCLAIMER

The information in this book and my videos has not been evaluated by the Food & Drug Administration or any other medical body.

I am not a doctor.

I do not aim to diagnose, treat, cure or prevent any illness or disease.

The information found in this book and my videos should be regarded as advice and opinions based on my experience and research.

All my information is shared for educational purposes only and should not be interpreted as medical advice.

You must consult your doctor before acting on any content in this book or videos, especially if you are pregnant, nursing, taking medication, or have a medical condition.

LEGAL DISCLAIMER

1. Introduction

This disclaimer governs the use of this book. [By using this book, you accept this disclaimer in full. I ask you to agree to this disclaimer before you can access the book.] No part of this book may be reproduced in any written, electronic, recording, or photocopying without written permission of the publisher or author. All trademarks are the exclusive property of JayCampbell.com

2. Credit

This disclaimer was created using an SEQ Legal template.

3. No advice

The book contains information about therapeutic peptides. The information is not advice and should not be treated as such. You must not rely on the information in the book as an alternative to medical advice from an appropriately qualified professional. If you have any specific questions about any matter, you should consult an appropriately qualified medical professional. If you think you may be suffering from any medical condition you should seek immediate medical attention. You should never delay seeking medical advice, disregard medical advice, or discontinue medical treatment because of information in this book

4. No representations or warranties

To the maximum extent permitted by applicable law and subject to section 6 below, we exclude all representations, warranties, undertakings and guarantees relating to the book. Without prejudice to the generality of the foregoing paragraph, we do not represent, warrant, undertake or guarantee: that the information in the book is correct, accurate, complete or non- misleading; that the use of the guidance in the book will lead to any particular outcome or result.

5. Limitations and exclusions of liability

The limitations and exclusions of liability set out in this section and elsewhere in this disclaimer: are subject to section 6 below; and govern all liabilities arising under the disclaimer or in relation to the book, including liabilities arising in contract, in tort (including negligence) and for breach of statutory duty. I will not be liable to you in respect of any losses arising out of any event or events beyond my reasonable control. I will not be liable to you in respect of any business losses, including without limitation loss of or damage to profits, income, revenue, use, production, anticipated savings, business, contracts, commercial opportunities or goodwill. I will not be liable to you in respect of any loss or corruption of any data, database or software. I will not be liable to you in respect of any special, indirect or consequential loss or damage.

6. Exceptions

Nothing in this disclaimer shall: limit or exclude my liability for death or personal injury resulting from negligence; limit or exclude my liability for fraud or fraudulent misrepresentation; limit any of my liabilities in any way that is not permitted under applicable law; or exclude any of my liabilities that may not be excluded under applicable law.

7. Severability

If a section of this disclaimer is determined by any court or other competent authority to be unlawful and/or unenforceable, the other sections of this disclaimer continue in effect.

If any unlawful and/or unenforceable section would be

lawful or enforceable if part of it were deleted, that part will be deemed to be deleted, and the rest of the section will continue in effect.

8. Law and jurisdiction

This disclaimer will be governed by and construed in accordance with law in the United States of America, and any disputes relating to this disclaimer will be subject to the exclusive jurisdiction of the courts of the United States of America.

9. Affiliate Disclosure

Some links to various products found inside this book contain affiliate links. If you make a purchase after clicking a link, I may receive a commission. This commission comes at no charge to you.

10. My details

In this disclaimer, "my" means (and "I" refers to) Jay Campbell (Playa Del Carmen, Mexico) and/or any future addresses, temporary or permanent.

CHAPTER 1
WHAT ARE THERAPEUTIC PEPTIDES?

At their simplest, peptides are biological compounds made up of two or more amino acids.

Each of us naturally produces a wide variety of peptides as part of our normal bodily function and regulation.

As we age and expose ourselves to different diets (i.e., GMO-processed foods), physical and mental changes, and environmental stressors and contaminants like endocrine disrupting chemicals (EDCs)[3], the production of these peptides decreases.

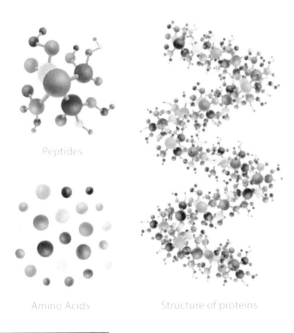

Peptides

Amino Acids

Structure of proteins

---

[3] http://pepbk.co/EDCs

As a result, our cellular processes become increasingly inefficient.

Peptides are different from proteins in that proteins are larger and usually cannot spontaneously rearrange into different structures.

It is their ability to chemically rearrange that enables therapeutic peptides to unlock the power of your body to heal itself.

As a revolutionary new form of regenerative medicine, peptides can be used to treat many chronic or acute conditions.

From ultimate health optimization to treating chronic diseases in people older than 40, these amazing compounds can improve, if not completely fix, many of the most common ailments so many people experience.

And with over 800 peptide drugs in the clinical pipeline and 197 commercially available[4], there's the potential for them to become a $75 billion market worldwide by 2028.

Suffice it to say, they are the present and future of medicine!

---

[4] http://pepbk.co/PeptidesMarket

Why Are Peptides Important as Tools for Regenerative Healing?

Peptides are a widely variable group of molecules serving many purposes and functions in the human body.

As such, each peptide will exert one or more effects impacting one or more biological systems within the human body.

When you start adding peptides back into your regimen -- whether using naturally derived peptides or lab-synthesized peptides -- you can unlock the body's ability to heal itself on a cellular level.

What Can You Expect After Using Therapeutic Peptides?

As soon as a few weeks after starting a regimen, you can expect potentially dramatic physiologic changes such as:

- *Faster rate of healing in soft tissue traumas like sprains, strains, or tears in ligament or tendons*

- *Increased short- and long-term memory*

- *Lower body fat and increased lean muscle tissue*

- *Stronger immunity against bioweapons and*

environmental toxins

Because peptides mimic our natural cellular behavior, they often have the potential to offer targeted treatments with fewer side effects.

This is because peptides are given in much smaller doses.

Whereas common medications are dispensed in doses measured in milligrams (mg), peptides are often dosed in micrograms (mcg) or even 1/1000th of that amount.

A Brief History on Peptides in Medicine

Believe it or not, peptides have been actively used in medicine for the past 100 years[5]:

> *"Starting about a century ago (World War I), the advent of the modern drug era came with pioneering therapeutic compounds like the opiate morphine and the cyclic peptide penicillin, followed in the early 1920s by the (poly)peptide insulin."*

---

[5] http://pepbk.co/History

However, small nonpeptide molecules were much easier to manufacture and administer for the pharmaceutical industry, which is why they were favored over peptides.

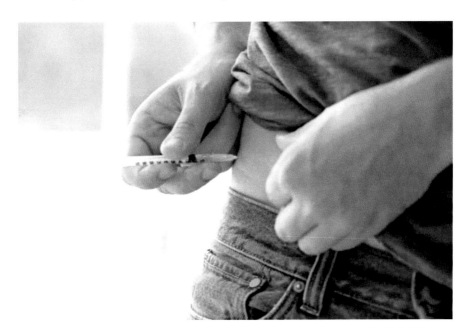

But this quickly worked against them and combined with the cost needed to bring one to the market alongside increasingly strict regulations, alternative solutions were needed[6]:

> "Fewer new drugs make it to the market and the patent protection of current blockbuster drugs is deteriorating, with a resulting drainage of the drug pipelines.
>
> All this may ultimately push the pharmaceutical

---

[6] http://pepbk.co/History

industry towards a new frontier in modern drug development."

Most interestingly, peptides have also been sought out as an alternative to antibodies[7]:

"Antibodies excel at target binding and PPI (protein-protein interaction) disruption with potency and specificity.

However, they carry certain liabilities, including an inability to access intracellular targets, poor tissue penetration, complex manufacturing and storage, immunogenic potential, and limitations to targets of sufficiently poor homology in host animals for B cell reactivity."

Why Are Therapeutic Peptides So Versatile?

Peptides are heavily used by doctors who focus on health optimization as they have a vested interest in providing the ultimate care for their patients.

The versatility of therapeutic peptides means they can help the body repair itself in many exciting ways.

---

[7] http://pepbk.co/AntibodiesAlternative

1. Therapeutic Peptides Treat NUMEROUS Conditions

Just look at this list from Concierge MD[8], a private doctor who uses therapeutic peptides to heal and enhance the human body:

- *Increasing bone strength and density*

- *Supporting joints*

- *Supporting a healthy libido*

- *Reducing erectile dysfunction*

- *Increasing muscle strength*

- *Improving sleep*

- *Boosting energy levels*

- *Supporting enhanced mood*

And that's just the tip of the iceberg.

You can also gain lean muscle, slow down aging, strengthen the immune system, increase IQ, lose stubborn body fat, and treat major diseases such as chronic inflammation, Alzheimer's, traumatic brain injury, and much more!

---

[8] http://pepbk.co/TreatableConditions

2. Therapeutic Peptides Can Be Administered In Several Ways

While each peptide will have an "optimal" form of delivery, there are several methods for administering them.

You can inject them subcutaneously[9] or intramuscularly[10].

A select few of them can even be taken as an oral formulation, like the muscle-building agent 5-Amino 1MQ[11].

3. Therapeutic Peptides Can Be Created Naturally or Synthetically

Many of the peptides discussed in this book are naturally produced by the body and resultantly produce very few side effects.

Other peptides can be synthetically created in a lab.

Many leading research teams have worked tirelessly to make them in a way that is both efficient and cost-effective.

---

[9] http://pepbk.co/SubQInjection
[10] http://pepbk.co/IMInjection
[11] http://pepbk.co/5-Amino1MQ

Important Things to Note About Using Therapeutic Peptides

Obviously, I believe in the power of therapeutic peptides.

But I'm not selling miracle water here.

As much as they can do for you, there are some things they cannot do.

It is important you have the right expectations before you grab a peptide vial and a syringe.

1. Therapeutic Peptides are NOT Instant Cures for Health Problems

In this age of big pharma advertising, many people have been conditioned with the expectation of near-instant results in medicine and healthcare.

If you've ever taken Adderall (mixed amphetamine salts), you know what I mean.

Shortly after dosing the medication, the person experiences instant alertness, increased energy, better focus, and so on.

That might sound like a good thing if you only look at half the story.

Any compound that has such an immediate effect is simply hiding the negative underlying state.

Popping amphetamines such as Adderall will allow you to stay awake, focused, and productive for days.

But the lack of sleep one experiences will eventually drive them into a state of psychosis and extract a heavy physical toll.

The reality of medicine is ultimately no different than anything else:

You need to devote time and work to get positive results, noticeable improvements, and fundamental changes for your body and your health.

Whether it is going to the gym regularly for six months to see real progress in your physique or being disciplined with nutrition for months to see real sustainable fat loss, TRUE fundamental progress in your state of health is a marathon and not a sprint.

There are exceptions to this rule, such as the nootropic peptides Selank[12] and Semax[13], which can be used for short periods of time (and rare situations) to heighten your mental performance.

But exceptions do not disprove the rule.

---

[12] http://pepbk.co/Selank
[13] http://pepbk.co/Semax

DO NOT use therapeutic peptides with the expectation of a quick fix!

To further illustrate, we can discuss the utilization of a peptide such as BPC-157[14] for healing a soft tissue injury.

Some people will report feeling a substantial improvement in less than a week after using BPC-157 once a day.

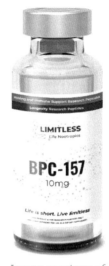

Image courtesy of Limitless Nootropics

The individual may feel better, and healing may indeed be taking place.

At the same time, the damaged tissue **is not** fully recovered and stabilized to a point where you would want to put it back under full load (which is likely what triggered the injury in the first place).

So even though you may feel better, you still need to use common sense and give your body time to fully heal.

In this instance, one should keep all physical activity involving the damaged area low, slowly increasing

---

[14] http://pepbk.co/BPC-157

range of motion (in said area) regardless of how quickly the healing process appears to be occurring.

2. Your State of Health Will Most Likely Dictate the Effect of Therapeutic Peptides

This is another important piece of the puzzle, especially when it comes to anti-aging protocols involving therapeutic peptides.

These types of peptides should come with the expectation of not experiencing significantly noticeable effects.

For instance, let's say you are periodically using Epitalon[15] or Pinealon as a fully optimized individual.

You wouldn't expect to see immediate or noticeable effects from periodic cycles of either of these compounds.

Why?

Because their purpose is to promote optimization at the cellular level to fight against cellular degradation over time.

This cellular degradation **leads to inflammation[16]**, which ultimately gives rise to multiple diseases

---

[15] http://pepbk.co/Epitalon
[16] http://pepbk.co/InflammatoryMarkers

associated with aging.

So how is this relevant to the state of a person's health and the perceived and actual results of effective therapeutic peptide use?

It is commonly believed the more optimized someone is, the better they will respond to peptide therapy.

Ironically, in some cases, the effects of a therapy are much more apparent in someone who is less optimized.

This is especially true when it comes to acute responses.

The more optimized one is, the more effectively their body will respond to the use of peptides in addressing an injury.

Yet the less optimized person may experience a more significant PERCEIVED effect, even if their body cannot respond to the therapy as effectively.

Therefore, it takes a greater degree of change for the effect of a treatment to be perceived.

Furthermore, people are generally better at noticing gradual changes instead of "static" changes.

If you were to wear a necklace every day for several

months, you would eventually reach a point where you don't "feel" it on your skin anymore.

The stimuli of the necklace on your skin becomes so commonplace, you lose conscious awareness of the necklace being worn.

This is where things get interesting: If you take the necklace off, the LACK of sensation is suddenly very noticeable.

This is admittedly a deep dive into psychology, but imperative to understand if you are using therapeutic peptides (or any other form of medication).

3. Watch Out for the Placebo Effect

Everyone reading this book has likely heard of and potentially experienced the placebo effect.

But just in case you haven't, here is verywellmind's definition[17] of what it is:

> *"The placebo effect is defined as a phenomenon in which some people experience a benefit after the administration of an inactive "look-alike" substance or treatment.*
>
> *The more a person expects the treatment to work, the more likely they are to exhibit a placebo*

---

[17] http://pepbk.co/Placebo

response.

This is due to the observer being the creator of their reality."

While the placebo effect can generate a very real and measurable physiological response due to an individual's own expectations, this is a double-edged sword.

The placebo effect may enhance your experience and make you feel instantly better.

On the other hand, you could feel as if you are experiencing negative side effects which aren't physiologically realistic given the peptide(s) being used.

Online forums and peptide communities are rife with people reporting all sorts of exaggerated placebo-induced side effects.

That's the problem with the placebo effect: it's a product of your own expectations.

If an individual went into the experience with a negative outlook or a high degree of anxiety, the smallest feedback supporting their initial outlook gets rapidly and negatively magnified from a psychological perspective.

This directly ties in with the importance of intelligently tracking every detail of your therapeutic peptide use if you want to be successful.

One can fall victim to the placebo effect, as well as have a lack of self- awareness of their physical state at any given moment.

Understanding this is a fact of life, and to make your usage of peptides as effective as possible, I recommend detailed tracking of your usage and results.

This ensures your expectations are aligned with the reality of your expected outcomes.

CHAPTER 2
THE TOP 10 MISTAKES I SEE PEOPLE MAKE WHEN STARTING PEPTIDES

Even though peptides have been used for over a hundred years, it's still extremely difficult to find high-quality information regarding their usage.

Because of this obvious fact, I strongly recommend anyone who wants to use them do their own research.

This is usually where things go wrong.

Using peptides is not as simple as following some Reddit poster's dosage recommendations.

You need to really know what you're doing.

I've consulted with hundreds of men and women personally (and hundreds of thousands via the internet) on the usage of therapeutic peptides and I often see the same mistakes over and over.

By avoiding these crucial mistakes, you will be on the fast track to seeing noticeable results.

1. Buying from a Non-Reputable Research Chemical Company

If possible, you should source your peptides from a

doctor's prescription.

This ensures the peptide is pharmaceutical grade and likely coming from the doctor's preferred compound pharmacy.

Because many peptides are becoming more restricted by the FDA for various reasons[18], it is critically important you vet where you are purchasing your peptides.

For that reason alone, I source all my peptides from (and recommend) **Limitless Life Nootropics**[19].

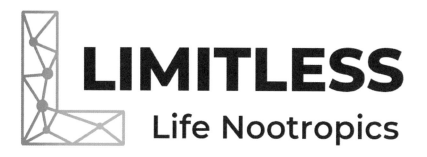

I know the owner personally[20] and am also familiar with their raw materials supplier, supply chain and manufacturing process.

Make sure you use code Jay15 to take 15% off your purchase.

[18] http://pepbk.co/PeptideSuppression
[19] http://pepbk.co/LimitlessLifeNootropics
[20] http://pepbk.co/ChristopherMercer

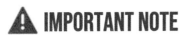

⚠ IMPORTANT NOTE

There are many non-reputable research chemical companies that manufacture their peptides in **non-sterile environments**.

Be very discerning and avoid buying from these companies at all costs.

2. Purchasing Peptides Without Also Purchasing Bacteriostatic Water

If you are sourcing your peptides from a research chemical company, you must also purchase sterile or bacteriostatic water[21] in order to reconstitute the peptide for storing in a refrigerated area afterwards.

3. Purchasing Peptides Without Also Acquiring the Proper Insulin Syringes

When one intends to be successful using peptides, all necessary ancillary equipment must be thought out and acquired at the same time.

One can purchase insulin syringes rather easily from Amazon[22] or various other online sellers.

These have a smaller gauge (thickness) than other

---

[21] http://pepbk.co/LLN-BacteriostaticWater
[22] http://pepbk.co/Syringes

needles.

4. Not Understanding How to Reconstitute Your Peptide with Bacteriostatic Water

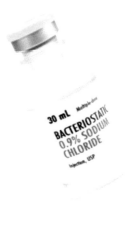

It is extremely important to understand how to withdraw bacteriostatic water and then inject it into your peptide vial without damaging the peptide.

This is a very simple process once understood.

It's a lot easier to do when you use a good calculator.

One that I created can be found here[23].

---

[23] http://pepbk.co/PeptideCalculator

> ### ⚠ IMPORTANT NOTE
>
> Understanding how to withdraw bacteriostatic water while simultaneously injecting it into the peptide vial (without damaging the active ingredient of the peptide) is a process known as *reconstitution*.
>
> The reconstitution process is critically important to learn when one starts out using peptides.
>
> A very good video tutorial demonstrating proper reconstitution technique can be found **here**[24].

5. Starting Peptides Without Understanding Proper Injection Procedure (i.e., Injecting Subcutaneously)

Injecting peptides is a simple process when one understands how to inject subcutaneously.

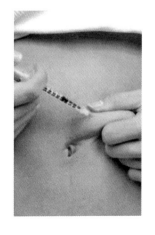

This is normally done in the lower abdominal area around the midsection where there is excess fat tissue.

---

[24] http://pepbk.co/HowToReconstitute

There are many videos online that demonstrate proper injection procedure for injections of peptides both **intramuscularly (IM)**[25] and **subcutaneously (subQ)**[26].

6. Not Understanding Proper Dosing and the Difference Between Milligram (mg) and Microgram (mcg)

It can be difficult to understand how to properly dose and inject your peptide.

Especially when vials of peptides come in different sizes and amounts (ex. 5mg, 10mg, 2mg, etc.)

You also must account for varying sizes of insulin syringes.

When at all possible, I recommend using 1ML syringes.

There are several tools to help clarify dosing, but I highly recommend using my **Peptide Calculator**[27] to convert from MG to MCG when preparing your dosing strategy.

---

[25] http://pepbk.co/IMInjection
[26] http://pepbk.co/SubQInjection
[27] http://pepbk.co/PeptideCalculator

7. Not Understanding the Role of Nutrition and Exercise in Attaining Results

Peptides won't do much for those who aren't already living a fully optimized lifestyle[28].

If you are obese, untrained (poorly conditioned), and not eating a clean diet (living insulin controlled), peptides will do very little if anything for you.

Before you start using peptides, I strongly recommend you first focus on cleaning up your diet, dropping body fat[29] (lowering inflammation), and starting a regular exercise program[30] (a combination of resistance and cardio-vascular training).

An excellent nutritional lifestyle to utilize is intermittent fasting.

My books *The Metabolic Blowtorch Diet*[31] and *Guaranteed Shredded*[32] are excellent resources for both newbies and advanced users to learn how to optimize fat loss protocols for maximum results.

---

[28] http://pepbk.co/DialingInYourLifestyle
[29] http://pepbk.co/FatLossStack
[30] http://pepbk.co/PMFTraining
[31] http://pepbk.co/TheMBTD
[32] http://pepbk.co/GuaranteedShredded

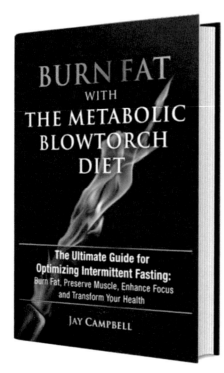 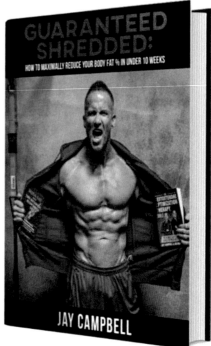

Becoming hormonally optimized first is also a great idea, as optimized testosterone levels can only enhance peptide utilization and results.

Towards the end of this book, you'll find out more about my therapeutic testosterone course (**TOT Decoded**[33]) to better understand whether you're suffering from a hormonal deficiency.

---

[33] http://pepbk.co/TOTDecoded

8. Having Unrealistic Expectations When Using Peptides

Peptides are not a magic bullet.

Once you have identified the specific reason you want to use a peptide, it's important to choose a peptide that addresses your problem.

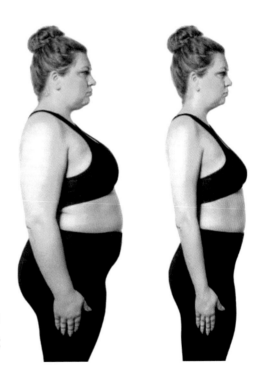

You must then create a peptide protocol that will work for you as an individual.

Is your condition acute (short-term) or chronic (sustained)?

Knowing the difference, what is your game plan?

How long will your cycle be?

How will you judge whether your peptide protocol was successful or not?

Outlining your expectations in advance will keep them within the realm of reality.

It also provides you with the most important element: A path to consistently measure and evaluate your progress.

9. Not Being Hormonally Optimized

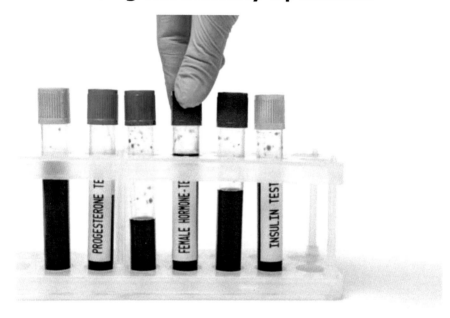

If a man or woman is already hormonally optimized, peptides will work in much greater synergy than for someone who is not.

Imagine your biological systems as a symphony orchestra.

If one part of your biological system isn't as finely tuned as the others, you won't get the same result.

Because many peptides work by improving and optimizing natural growth hormone release, having optimized hormones (such as testosterone and estradiol) only enhances the synergy between the two.

I elaborate about this in a 11-minute video[34] I highly recommend viewing.

10. Not Understanding the Differences Between Various Peptide Delivery Systems

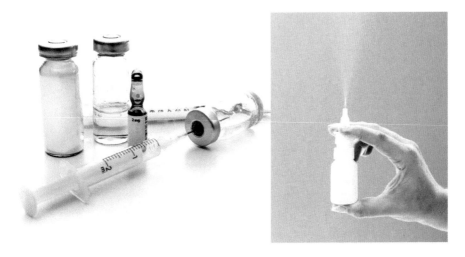

There are many misinformed doctors and online experts recommending peptides to be used "orally", "intra-nasally", and through other delivery systems.

It is critically important to be aware that not all routes of administration are equal and not all methods of administration produce the same effect.

Most peptides are poorly absorbed orally and intra-

[34] http://pepbk.co/PeptidesBeforeHormones

nasally (some exceptions apply) and taking them this way will drastically limit their therapeutic effects.

 IMPORTANT NOTE

Subcutaneous (SubQ) or shallow intramuscular (IM) injection are the highest impact delivery systems for virtually all peptides.

CHAPTER 3
THE BEST PEPTIDES FOR FAT LOSS

Everyone has different goals when it comes to using peptides.

Some people are looking to improve their body while others are looking to improve their mind.

These next several chapters will examine the different peptides and their numerous biological effects.

Take specific notes so you can come back to the peptides that fit your individual goals.

One of the most common desired outcomes when using therapeutic peptides is fat loss.

And why would it not be when nearly 45% of the United States is now labeled "clinically obese" according to the latest data[35] from the CDC?

I've experimented with all the fat loss peptides in existence personally and have also used them on my private coaching clients.

After nearly two decades of gathering results, I'm ready to present the eight best fat-burning peptides in existence.

---

[35] http://pepbk.co/StateOfObesity

Ipamorelin

Ipamorelin[36] was one of the first peptides I ever used, and also one of the few worthy enough to get a mention in both **The TOT Bible**[37] and **Living A Fully Optimized Life**[38].

Ipamorelin is a GHRP (growth hormone releasing peptide), which means it produces a pulse that mimics your body's natural growth hormone release.

It does so via increased signaling to the pituitary gland and inhibition of a hormone called somatostatin, which "tells" your body to lower its output of (endogenous) growth hormone production.

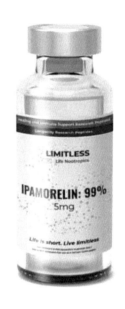

Ipamorelin is unique because it will ONLY target growth hormone without affecting other bodily hormones such as prolactin or cortisol.

You also don't see increased production of the appetite-stimulating hormone ghrelin, which helps keep hunger at bay while fasting.

---

[36] http://pepbk.co/Ipamorelin
[37] http://pepbk.co/TheTOTBible
[38] http://pepbk.co/LAFOL

Other secondary fat loss benefits include deeper sleep, improved muscle growth, and slight cognition-enhancing effects.

Ipamorelin is recommended as the best "introductory" peptide for fat loss if increased natural (i.e., endogenous) growth hormone production is desired.

Recommended Dosage

This is my optimal protocol designed to give you the best Ipamorelin dose for fat loss (and potentially muscle gain when combined with above maintenance calorie consumption):

 IPAMORELIN RECOMMENDED DOSAGE

200-300 mcg injected subcutaneously one to three times a day.

It is recommended to cycle Ipamorelin for no longer than 8 weeks with an equal amount of time off for maximum efficacy.

However, I provide some additional details in **The TOT Bible**[39] for different use cases:

---

[39] http://pepbk.co/TheTOTBible

*"Some users inject Ipamorelin **30-45 minutes before training** to take advantage of the hGH (human growth hormone) pulse and maximize both training intensity and fat loss.*

Most users will see body composition changes with 300 mcg, once or twice per day, over a 3-month period (or longer).

*For women especially, an **injection of 200-300 mcg immediately before bed** can produce dramatic fat loss and improved body composition in less than 3 months (when combined with resistance training, cardiovascular training and insulin-controlled living)."*

It was that exact dosage of Ipamorelin I used with my wife Monica to radically alter her physique when we first started dating in 2012.

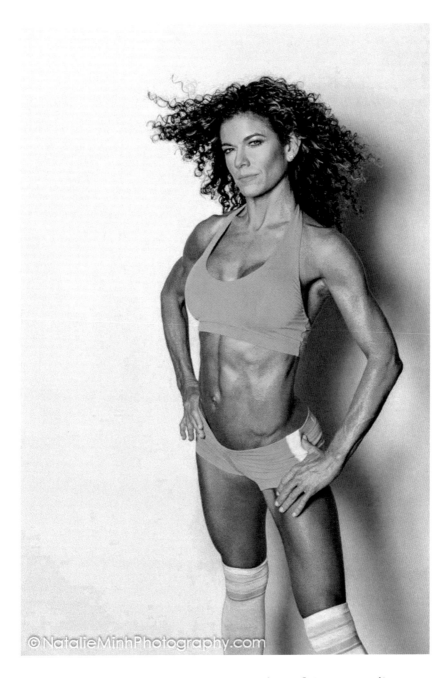

The image shown is after 8 months of Ipamorelin usage
when Monica was 41 years old.

(Please note Monica had given birth to 3 children prior to that photo.

She is living proof peptides can make dramatic changes to body composition when combined with proper nutrition, intelligent training and hormonally optimized living.)

And before I receive any feedback the image is of Monica from 10 years ago, this image is from late January 2023 where Monica is now 51 years young.

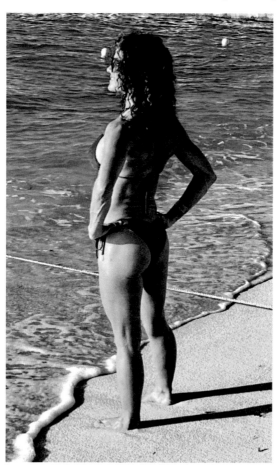

Tesofensine

Tesofensine[40] is not technically a peptide but is one of the hottest new fat loss drugs on the market.

I would be doing it a massive disservice by not including it in this book.

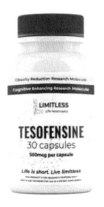

(You can purchase Tesofensine from Limitless Life Nootropics here[41]. Remember to use code JAY15 for 15% off.)

Tesofensine is a triple monoamine reuptake inhibitor originally designed as a new class of antidepressant.

It first emerged as a treatment for Alzheimer's but ultimately was orphaned.

By mere accident, a major side effect of this drug in clinical trials was significant weight loss without additional exercise or dietary interventions.

How does it work?

• *It stops dopamine reuptake, which reduces the feeling of mental cravings*

---

[40] http://pepbk.co/Tesofensine
[41] http://pepbk.co/LLN-Tesofensine

- *It stops serotonin reuptake, which reduces the PHYSICAL need of hunger*

- *It stops noradrenaline reuptake, which increase your basal metabolic rate*

Tesofensine induces twice the amount of weight loss compared to existing anti-obesity medications in head-on clinical trials (and keeps it off).

It also dramatically increases the production of BDNF[42] (Brain-Derived Neurotrophic Factor), a growth factor expressed in your brain that enhances cognition and the ability to achieve a flow state.

This is also on top of the fat loss effects it provides as a metabolic uncoupler over time.

And did I mention it comes in a capsule form you only have to take once a day in the morning?

Tesofensine is an all-in-one fat-destroying compound that is the closest thing to a "Holy Grail of Fat Loss".

Recommended Dosage

I want to emphasize again that Tesofensine comes in the form of a convenient capsule/tablet.

---

[42] http://pepbk.co/BDNF

TESOFENSINE RECOMMENDED DOSAGE

One 0.5 mg dosage first thing in the morning while fasted (to cross the blood brain barrier maximizing absorption) is all that is required.

An obese individual may need to go up to two tablets (1 mg total) per day, although the lead author of the pivotal 2008 clinical trial, Dr. Arne Astrup, insists 0.5 mg is good enough[43]:

> *"Twelve percent of the 0.5-mg group did not complete the study, as compared with 29% of the 1.0-mg group and 25% of the placebo group.*
>
> *Of the patients who dropped out of the study's 1.0-mg arm, 20.4% did so because of adverse effects, compared with a combined average of 8% in the other groups.*
>
> *Dr. Astrup suggested that the optimal dose for Tesofensine may be 0.5 mg.*
>
> *'There's no reason to pursue [a potential dose of 1.0 mg],' he noted, 'because it doesn't produce much more weight loss, but [it] increases*

---

[43] http://pepbk.co/TesofensineClinicalTrial

problems.'"

Keep in mind the recommended dosing strategy for Tesofensine exists despite its abnormally long half-life of 234 hours (~9-10 days).

It most likely explains why people still feel satiated a week after Tesofensine use is stopped but then gradually feel hungry again.

⚠ IMPORTANT NOTE

It has been reported by select users that Tesofensine is so strong in its stimulatory effect it can potentially disturb sleep.

It is my opinion that previous users of SSRI medications are the most susceptible due to the rewiring of their various brain pathways.

For this reason, it is recommended to never dose after 10 AM.

Tesamorelin

Tesamorelin[44], unlike its relative Ipamorelin, is known as a GHRH (growth hormone releasing hormone).

GHRHs work by stimulating your brain's pituitary gland to increase the production and secretion of human growth hormone.

The good news is Tesamorelin stimulates GHRH receptors just as well as the GHRH naturally produced by your body.

It does this without inducing insulin resistance or affecting the production of bodily hormones, like how Ipamorelin works.

Thanks to bodybuilders and their willingness to experiment with anything that gives them a competitive edge, we know Tesamorelin directly leads to fat loss in the abdominal region.

This ultimately enhances the vascularity and appearance of one's abs.

How?

Out of all the fat loss peptides, Tesamorelin specifically targets visceral fat around the abdominal area -- the closest we've ever come to spot fat reduction.

---

[44] http://pepbk.co/Tesamorelin

Secondary benefits include enhanced cognition, slight muscle gain, and lower triglyceride readings.

Unfortunately, Tesamorelin is a prescription medication meant to treat lipodystrophy in HIV patients.

Lipodystrophy is an abnormal distribution of body fat that selectively accumulates in the trunk region.

This medical condition produces hard visceral belly fat which is difficult to burn off.

If you are one of the lucky few individuals who gets their hands on pharma grade Tesamorelin, it's your best choice for specifically getting rid of stubborn body fat in your trunk region.

Recommended Dosage

Having used Tesamorelin myself to maintain single-digit body fat levels year-round, and recommended its use to numerous private coaching clients, I have precise recommendations for dosing Tesamorelin.

The optimal dose of Tesamorelin for fat loss has previously been described in my book, **Guaranteed Shredded**[45]:

---

[45] http://pepbk.co/GuaranteedShredded

TESAMORELIN RECOMMENDED DOSAGE

1 mg injected subcutaneously at night before bed (but at least 90 minutes after your last meal), and 1 mg injected subcutaneously upon waking up in the morning (ideally before fasted cardio or exercising).

If you're going to inject Tesamorelin only once per day, inject it at night as recommended above.

With my female clients, a once-a-day injection of 1 mg of Tesamorelin works wonders for improving polyphasic sleep and night-time growth hormone production.

Using the "five days on, two days off"[46] cycle is popular, which involves injecting 1 mg subcutaneously in the morning fasted before cardio.

I personally recommend people use Tesamorelin for no longer than 60 days in a row before taking a similarly long break to cycle off.

For men and women who are already living a clean, low inflammation lifestyle, it normally takes four to six weeks to observe noticeable changes in body

---

[46] http://pepbk.co/HowToUsePeptides

composition (i.e., increase in lean muscle mass, decrease in visceral body fat, etc.).

If you are a person who is 20% body fat or higher, your results will not be as noticeable as someone with significantly less body fat.

I recommend you temper your expectations accordingly.

AOD-9604

AOD-9604[47] is a synthetic modification of a very specific region within human growth hormone that is solely responsible for accelerating the metabolism of fat.

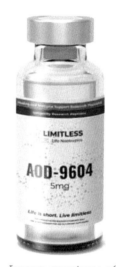

Surprisingly, in select clinical studies, AOD-9604 has been shown to be better than growth hormone itself at inhibiting fat production and promoting fat breakdown.

Image courtesy of Limitless Nootropics

And thanks to its lack of interaction with growth hormone receptors, it doesn't cause insulin resistance.

---

[47] http://pepbk.co/AOD-9604

However, despite an excellent safety profile in humans, clinical trials in mostly obese and comorbid patient population groups did not show a meaningful difference in weight loss compared to placebo.

Thankfully, numerous biohackers have taken it upon themselves to experiment with AOD9604 and swear by its fat loss effects.

That includes yours truly, especially when used in combination with another peptide. More on that later.

Therefore, AOD9604 is an excellent fat loss peptide for increasing fat metabolism and inhibiting fat production.

Recommended Dosage

Although there is insufficient data to recommend an optimal AOD-9604 dose, I have personally used this peptide alongside Semaglutide[48] with phenomenal success.

But using AOD-9604 alone, you can go one of two ways:

---

[48] http://pepbk.co/SemaglutideAndAOD-9604

AOD-9604 RECOMMENDED DOSAGE

- *A once-a-day subcutaneous injection of 300 mcg, preferably in the morning while fasted (before cardio, or 1 hour before your first meal)*

- *A twice-a-day subcutaneous injection of 250 mcg, once in the morning before fasted cardio (or at least 1 hour before your first meal) and once before bedtime (1-4 hours after your last meal).*

(Credit goes to Dr. William Seeds for recommending the second protocol)

You can do a cycle as short as six weeks or as long as six months with either method you choose, taking a one-week break to reset before beginning another cycle where necessary.

You can also choose to fast for three to four hours (or much longer if following my **Blowtorch Diet**[49] alternate day fasting program) after your first morning injection and see if a fasted state increases the rate of fat loss.

---

[49] http://pepbk.co/TheMBTD

You'll also get optimal results by injecting AOD-9604 into the "fattest" parts of your body, i.e., your midsection.

Make sure to give your chosen protocol at least three months of use to judge how effective AOD-9604 is at reaching your ideal body fat percentage.

(NOTE: While some peptide clinics endorse combining AOD-9604 with NAD+, I personally cannot vouch for this)

Finally, make sure you are storing your reconstituted AOD-9604 in your refrigerator.

It is recommended you finish the entire bottle within two to four weeks.

 IMPORTANT NOTE

How long do reconstituted peptides last in refrigeration?

It depends on who you ask, but most peptide formulators say that once a peptide is reconstituted and left inside a refrigerator for re-use, the efficacy of the peptide will last between 2 and 4 weeks.

Semaglutide

Semaglutide is a synthetic modification of a hormone peptide known as GLP-1 (glucagon-like peptide-1).

It's effectively the same molecule with a few minor adjustments[50].

This makes Semaglutide a GLP-1 receptor agonist, which is a technical way of saying the following:

> *"Semaglutide is part of a class of medications called GLP-1 receptor agonists, or glucagon-like peptide-1 receptor agonists.*
>
> *It increases insulin secretion, which is good for diabetes.*
>
> *At higher doses, **it acts on centers in the brain and suppresses appetite**.*
>
> *What this medicine does is help patients adhere to a reduced-calorie diet."*
>
> *- University of Alabama at Birmingham*

Semaglutide is an excellent peptide for helping to reduce body fat as it directly addresses the negative behavior of overeating via appetite suppression.

---

[50] http://pepbk.co/Semaglutide

Due to the dramatic weight loss seen in clinical trials spanning two years (making it almost as drastic as bariatric surgery), the FDA approved it in June 2021[51] *"for chronic weight management in adults with obesity who are overweight with at least one weight-related condition."*

Having used Semaglutide myself, I can attest to how free of hunger I felt when on it.

As a once-a-week peptide injection, adhering to the dosing schedule is not difficult.

Semaglutide, if you can get it via prescription or other means, will significantly suppress appetite.

 IMPORTANT NOTE

Tirzepatide, discussed next, offers noticeably stronger appetite suppression and metabolic uncoupling, thereby enhancing the rate of fat loss.

(Because of these two qualities, I like it more than Semaglutide)

---

[51] http://pepbk.co/SemaglutideFDA

Recommended Dosage

SEMAGLUTIDE RECOMMENDED DOSAGE

Dr. Rudolph Eberwein of **Medical Health Institute**[52] shared the following dosing protocol with me for using AOD9604 and Semaglutide simultaneously:

Semaglutide — start with a 0.25 mg subcutaneous injection once a week, increasing the dose every 4 weeks up to a maximum of 2.4 mg

AOD9604 — a subcutaneous injection of 300 mcg once a day, going as high as 500-600 mcg preferably upon awakening while fasted.

(NOTE: While Dr. Eberwein states most of his obese patients already see results within the 0.25 mg – 1.25 mg range for Semaglutide, healthy individuals may need something different.

I have found through my own experimentation that 0.4-0.5 mg is more than enough to elicit optimal results.)

As both peptides are injectable solutions, you will need

---

[52] http://pepbk.co/MedicalHealthInstitute

to rotate subcutaneous injection sites for best results.

Tirzepatide

Tirzepatide[53] is what many consider to be the successor to Semaglutide[54] when it comes to superior weight loss and appetite suppression.

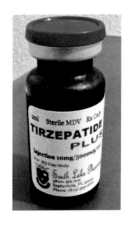

This peptide was developed by Eli Lilly and is marketed under the brand name "Mounjaro."

Tirzepatide is a synthetic modification of a hormone peptide known as glucose-dependent insulinotropic peptide (GIP), which carries out the following functions when attached to its receptor:

- *Induces insulin secretion*

- *Increases insulin sensitivity*

- *Improves lipid metabolism and triglyceride clearance*

- *Lowers bodyweight*

---

[53] http://pepbk.co/Tirzepatide
[54] http://pepbk.co/SemaglutideAndAOD-9604

Not only does Tirzepatide target GIP's receptors, but it also targets the same receptors of glucagon-like peptide-1 (GLP-1) as Semaglutide does.

GLP-1's biological functions[55] are highly similar yet somewhat different from those of GIP:

- *Suppresses glucagon secretion*

- *Blunts appetite (giving you the feeling of being full)*

- *Stimulates insulin release from pancreas to lower blood glucose levels*

- *Delays gastric emptying*

So, while Semaglutide only targeted GLP-1 receptors, Tirzepatide goes after the receptors of both GLP-1 AND GIP.

And across numerous Phase 3 trials[56], Tirzepatide was superior to placebo and any other equivalent drug such as Semaglutide when faced head-to-head in both diabetic and non-diabetic obese patients.

Specifically, patients found themselves feeling much fuller and losing way more body weight within the same period.

---

[55] http://pepbk.co/GLP-1
[56] http://pepbk.co/TirzepatidePhase3Trials

Researchers also observed big reductions in glycosylated hemoglobin (HbA1c), and an equivalent (if not lower) severity and frequency of side effects in comparison to Semaglutide and other GLP-1 receptor agonists.

Due to Tirzepatide's status as a prescription drug, it is difficult to purchase online.

You must speak with a doctor who will write a script for you.

Not to mention Tirzepatide's hefty price tag of anywhere between $500 and $1,000 per month at the recommended weekly dose per standard instructions.

You may be able to offset some of the cost if you qualify through your insurance provider.

Recommended Dosage

 TIRZEPATIDE RECOMMENDED DOSAGE

For a healthy person (not obese) 2.5 mg injected subcutaneously once a week for a month (4 weeks total), and then increasing to 5 mg injected subcutaneously once per week for the second month.

For obese people in serious need of glycemic control due to diabetes, keep increasing the dose in 2.5 mg increments every four weeks but never exceed 15 mg injected subcutaneously once a week.

 IMPORTANT NOTE

Most healthy people experience dramatic results at just the weekly recommended dosage of 2.5 mg.

I recommend cycling it twice per year with an equal amount of time off in between use cycles.

MOTS-C

MOTS-C[57] is a naturally occurring peptide produced by the mitochondria in your cells.

It didn't receive much attention until several studies in obese mice showed it was able to replicate the positive health benefits of exercising without exercising!

The mechanism of a fat-burning peptide like MOTS-C is quite complicated.

It involves a lot of downstream biochemical cascade reactions that reduce fat accumulation.

MOTS-C can also improve insulin sensitivity, increase fat breakdown, boost your energy levels, and even enhance mitochondrial health[58].

Out of all the peptides to lose weight I've featured up until this point, MOTS-C is the most experimental.

I have personally noticed it doesn't have as much of an effect in people who are already lean (likely due to their already enhanced mitochondrial function).

Use MOTS-C if you possess higher levels of body fat and are willing to use a fat loss peptide without the scientific backing of the other peptides featured in

---

[57] http://pepbk.co/MOTS-C
[58] http://pepbk.co/OptimizeMitochondrialHealth

this book.

Recommended Dosage

I usually offer a blanket recommendation for dosing peptides, but I'm going to make an exception for MOTS-C.

Because truthfully, the best MOTS-C dose for enhanced fat loss and better endurance is still up in the air.

That's why I'm going to share various protocols suggested by some of the top peptide experts in the world...

MOTS-C RECOMMENDED DOSAGE

Ben Greenfield in his book Boundless[59]: 10 mg of MOTS-C injected once a week, ideally right before endurance exercise for the added mitochondrial benefit, can be repeated for up to 10 weeks in a row every year.

Dr. William Seeds in his book *Peptide Protocols*, Volume 1[60]: 5 mg of MOTS-C injected subcutaneously 3 times per week on a Monday-Wednesday-Friday schedule for 4-6 weeks, followed by a once-a-week dose of 5 mg for 4 weeks.

Dr. Rob Kominiarek[61]: 10 mg of MOTS-C injected subcutaneously into the abdomen once a week for 4 weeks straight, followed by a second 4-week cycle within a 12-month period.

Jay Campbell experimented with 2mg of MOTS-C every third day for two weeks and 5 mg all at once.

---

[59] http://pepbk.co/Boundless
[60] http://pepbk.co/PeptideProtocolsVol1
[61] http://pepbk.co/RenueHealth

I recommend using this peptide in the morning to avoid any potential disturbance of sleep patterns.

It has also been shown to provide a noticeable energy boost within 30 minutes of administration for some users.

And while I cannot confirm this 100%, some MOTS-C users claim the peptide degrades rapidly upon being reconstituted due to its high level of instability (50% at 2 hours and 90% at three hours).

For that reason, you might consider injecting the MOTS-C peptide immediately after it has been prepared.

5-Amino 1MQ

5-Amino 1MQ[62] (technically considered a small molecule) is the very last of the fat-burning ergogens I AM including in the book, but it is highly effective in many of its users.

5-Amino is a synthetic analog of a chemical called methylquinolinium (MQ) and was designed when scientists were looking for a NNMT (nicotinamide N-methyltransferase) inhibitor.

---

[62] http://pepbk.co/5-Amino1MQ

Without getting into the technical details, the NNMT enzymes slow down the metabolism of fat cells, making it a viable target for anti-obesity medications.

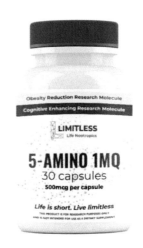

But restoration of fat burning, and fat breakdown are just some of the things 5-Amino 1MQ can do.

This wonder agent can also improve neuromuscular function and increase your ability to maximally contract your muscle fibers through the same mechanism of NNMT inhibition.

Having used it myself, I was able to put on 10 pounds of lean muscle in six weeks without changing my diet and training regimen or using other therapeutic peptides[63].

On top of reducing delayed onset muscle soreness (DOMS) after intense high-volume workouts, it has the bonus of lowering cellular senescence[64].

---

[63] http://pepbk.co/ListOfPeptides
[64] http://pepbk.co/SenescentCells

So what we have in effect is a "body recomposition agent" that aids in both maximal fat loss AND maximal muscle preservation.

5-Amino 1MQ is an excellent ergogen for maintaining and increasing muscle mass depending on whether you are eating calories at maintenance or in a caloric surplus.

Recommended Dosage

There isn't an established 5-Amino 1MQ dosage for either enhanced muscle growth and/or fat loss.

I have managed to find a dosing protocol that was most effective for my body recomposition goals.

 5-AMINO 1MQ RECOMMENDED DOSAGE

My optimal dose of 5-Amino 1MQ is 50 mg to 150 mg once a day with food in the form of a capsule for 20-30 days before taking a break for 1-2 weeks.

> ### ⚠ IMPORTANT NOTE
>
> In many users, 5-Amino 1MQ tends to become less effective if used for more than 8-12 weeks.
>
> I recommend cycling it twice per year with an equal amount of time off in between use cycles.

Due to 5-Amino's oil-solubility, I want to emphasize the importance of taking 5-Amino 1MQ with food for maximum absorption.

In my experience using 5-Amino 1MQ, I have found it works best with short 3–6-week dosing cycles.

One of the main reasons users like 5-Amino 1MQ is it doesn't have to be injected (subcutaneously or intramuscularly) as maximum benefits are attained from oral consumption.

This was understood when researchers at Texas Southern University determined the majority of 5-Amino was eliminated in the urine without any structural changes when given via injection.

Most peptide vendors will usually sell 5-Amino 1MQ in the form of 50 mg capsules, so you'll end up taking 1-3 capsules per day.

⚠ IMPORTANT NOTE

As with any supplement I recommend, start at the lower end of the dosing range and gradually work your way up.

Starting low and going slow to assess your individual tolerance is always the prudent course of action when starting most medications or supplements.

CHAPTER 4
THE BEST PEPTIDES FOR LONGEVITY

The best anti-aging peptides on the market have been extensively studied for decades.

The scientific literature available for each one is significant and overwhelmingly positive.

This is in sharp contrast to the many fat loss peptides[65] and nootropic peptides[66] that are backed by mostly animal studies and the anonymous testimonials of brave biohackers.

Due to the significant clinical research demonstrating the benefit of anti-aging peptides, it's only a matter of time before the mainstream healthcare industry is aware of them.

GHK-Cu

The copper peptide GHK-Cu[67] has a long history since its discovery in human blood in the early 1970s by the scientist Dr. Loren Pickart.

---

[65] http://pepbk.co/FatLossPeptides
[66] http://pepbk.co/NootropicPeptides
[67] http://pepbk.co/GHK-Cu

Dr Pickart is responsible for most published studies studying this molecule.

It is a complex formed by the tripeptide "GHK" and copper, an essential mineral for human health and the development of connective tissue.

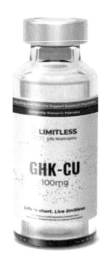

In its raw constituted form, it appears as a brilliant, shimmery bluish-purple color.

And as a naturally occurring peptide, its production in the human body fades with time.

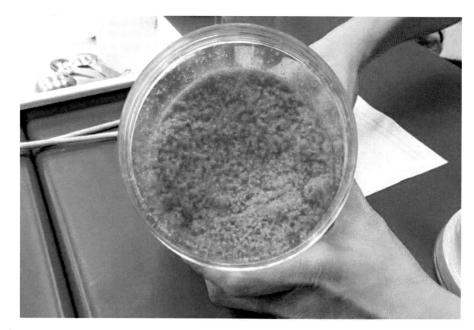

Not only is it a powerful antioxidant with anti-inflammatory properties, it also repairs damaged DNA via enhancing immunity against bacteria and viruses.

One of GHK-Cu's primary features is the acceleration of wound healing, primarily via the production of the protein collagen and the stimulation of new blood vessel growth (angiogenesis).

These two mechanisms, on top of stimulating production of the protein elastin, are why GHK-Cu is also an effective skin care agent[68].

Numerous human and animal trials have found GHK-Cu can:

- *Lower the formation of wrinkles*

- *Protect against ultraviolet (UV) radiation and damage*

- *Repair skin wounds and scars*

- *Improve skin elasticity and hydration*

- *Lower hyperpigmentation*

- *Reverse hair loss[69]*

GHK-Cu is the ONLY peptide listed in this book that

---

[68] http://pepbk.co/GHK-CuSkinCare
[69] http://pepbk.co/GHK-CuForHairLoss

functions best as a transdermal delivery system (i.e., a topical cream or serum).

If your goal with anti-aging is **specifically targeted towards slowing the appearance of aging in your skin and face**, I strongly recommend GHK-Cu as your primary option.

Recommended Dosage

GHK-Cu is extremely easy to use due to most formulations coming in the form of a cream or serum applied topically to the area of interest.

This holds true for treating aging skin or "red" skin from sunburn or age-related damage.

After cleansing your skin (usually by showering), apply a LIGHT amount of GHK-Cu cream or serum to the skin and gently massage it in for 5-10 seconds.

Apply just enough cream to barely cover the area of interest.

If you are using a 3% GHK-Cu formulation, this means using 2-4 pumps (0.21 mL – 0.81 mL) on average per application.

The more severe your injury, the more often you will have to apply GHK-Cu.

Reputable suppliers of GHK-Cu-based products such as creams and serums are currently in short supply.

As more become available, you might consider visiting **pepbk.co/GHK-CuProducts** to view my most up-to-date recommendation(s).

CJC-1295

Before I talk about this anti-aging peptide, I need to give a short background about human growth hormone (hGH)[70] because it is a core part of anti-aging medicine as a whole:

> *"Clinical studies have shown that low-dose growth hormone (GH) treatment for adults with GH deficiency changes the body composition by increasing muscle mass, decreasing fat mass, and increasing bone density and muscle strength.*
>
> *It also improves cardiovascular parameters (i.e., decrease of LDL cholesterol) and affects the quality of life without significant side effects"*
>
> *- Wikipedia[71]*

Just like GHK-Cu, natural hGH production decreases over time (a loss of roughly 14% every 10 years).

Many scientists/researchers believe injecting hGH is

---

[70] http://pepbk.co/hGH
[71] http://pepbk.co/hGHWikipedia

medically not viable for several reasons:

- *In some studies, it has been shown to reduce the body's natural production of hGH (potentially negatively affecting your pituitary gland's endogenous production)*

- *Higher dosage use over time increases the risk of insulin resistance*

- *Extremely expensive*

- *Usually only prescribed for VERY specific medical conditions, especially those focused on lack of normal hGH production at very young ages*

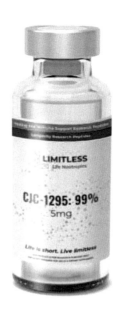

⚠ IMPORTANT NOTE

In my nearly two years of experience using pharmaceutical hGH from Pfizer (Genotropin) at surgically precise dosages (1-2 IU's taken in the morning Monday thru Friday) combined with Metformin[72] and living and eating "insulin controlled", I have experienced none of the theorized negative potential effects of using hGH.

Because of my personal experience dispelling the negative perceptions of hGH, it is my strong recommendation that if one can locate pharmaceutical grade hGH legally and can afford its use, it is preferable to peptides.

This is especially true for men and women who are 50 years or older.

You can read much more about hGH in this deeply informative article[73] on my website.

Let's briefly review the two types of anti-aging peptides helping us stimulate the pathways leading to hGH production, while only minimally affecting our body's natural means of producing and distributing hGH.

Growth hormone releasing hormone (GHRH):

---

[72] http://pepbk.co/Metformin
[73] http://pepbk.co/hGH

Responsible for the frequency and timing of the body's "pulses" that secrete hGH through increasing production of hGH-releasing cells (somatotropes) and the amount of hGH released by the cells.

Growth hormone releasing peptide (GHRP): Increases the size of the pulses by inhibiting somatostatin production to prevent inhibition of hGH release and promotes the release of more GHRH.

Smart experiential-based doctors know that combining both a GHRP and a GHRH is the best way to always maximize natural hGH production.

This brings us back to CJC-1295[74], a small fragment of naturally occurring GHRH responsible for increasing hGH production.

You'll normally see it labeled as including (or not including) a "drug affinity complex" (DAC) that gives the peptide a longer half-life in the body.

On top of the general positive health benefits of hGH described earlier, CJC-1295 can also:

- *Make your sleep deeper*

- *Accelerate your body's ability to heal wounds and injuries*

---

[74] http://pepbk.co/CJC-1295

- *Increase energy levels*

- *Lower inflammation*

- *Restore insulin sensitivity*

If you're looking to **improve your body composition** while optimizing metabolic health and heart health, CJC-1295 is a nice option and often used alongside Ipamorelin to enhance both of their effects.

Recommended Dosage

I'm still uncertain on what a good CJC-1295 dosing protocol in isolation would look like as I have only used it sparingly and in combination with Ipamorelin.

Here are some recommendations from experienced users...

CJC-1295 RECOMMENDED DOSAGE

One protocol from an integrative medicine specialist suggests *"injecting 0.10ml of a 2000 mcg/mL subcutaneously 5 out of 7 nights of the week before bedtime on an empty stomach for 6–8-week cycles."*

Dr. William Seeds uses the following protocols depending on which variation of CJC-1295 is being administered:

- *CJC-1295 WITHOUT DAC: A saturation dose of 100 mcg is typically used (1 mg/kg), as any higher dosage adds minimally to the pulse of GH released*

- *CJC-1295 WITH DAC: Twice a week at 100 mcg, OR 100 mcg daily (this dose works best for short-term treatment to elevate IGF1 above physiologic levels)*

Others have suggested anywhere from 200-350 mcg a week, but results may vary.

If you're new to peptides and you're wondering "What is DAC and why must I care?" listen closely as it does affect your dosage.

DAC (Drug Affinity Complex) is an extra ingredient prolonging the half-life of CJC-1295 (up to 8 days).

The *half-life* of any drug is defined as the amount of time it stays effective in your system.

If one uses CJC-1295 with DAC, its effects are extended up to two weeks after administration.

This is the reason for the variance in dosage recommendations.

Regardless of whether you choose CJC with or without DAC, Dr. Seeds recommends avoiding food consumption 30 minutes before use and 1.5 hours after using it.

This is in order to maintain optimal absorption as carb and fat consumption limits the drug's ability to cross the blood brain barrier which ultimately blunts growth hormone release.

Understanding this, my best advice is to take it either before bed on an empty stomach (thus improving sleep) or in the morning, fasted before your first meal.

Ipamorelin

Continuing the discussion of hGH, Ipamorelin[75] is a GHRP that differs greatly from other molecules in its class (Hexarelin, GHRP-2, etc.).

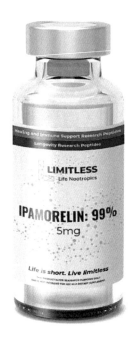

It ONLY targets hGH production/release and does not elevate the production of other hormones such as cortisol and prolactin, both of which reduce the breakdown of fat tissue at high levels.

Ipamorelin also does not touch the hunger hormone ghrelin, meaning your level of hunger will be reduced.

This is an absolute must if your primary goal is **reducing body fat**.

Ipamorelin is an excellent choice in combination with an intermittent fasting protocol like the one found in my advanced fat loss book *Guaranteed Shredded*[76].

Ipamorelin shares many of the positive health benefits as CJC-1295 but the other notable outcomes of Ipamorelin use include:

---

[75] http://pepbk.co/Ipamorelin
[76] http://pepbk.co/GuaranteedShredded

- *Better gut health*

- *Favorable effects on cognitive health*

- *Stronger bones*

- *Accelerated fat loss*

- *Decreased joint and muscle pain*

- *Enhanced workout recovery*

Ipamorelin is my favorite peptide when used in isolation due to its excellent sleep-improving and fat loss benefits combined with its minimal side effect profile.

As mentioned in the previous section of this book covering fat loss peptides, Ipamorelin is an amazing peptide for women due to its easy-to-follow strategy of taking one dose before bed.

It yields significant and noticeable results in a very minimum amount of time for most female users.

If you are looking to enhance its effect, it can be combined synergistically with CJC-1295 to provide both a GHRP and GHRH pulse together.

In theory and in practice, both peptides used together produce a stronger effect than if used in isolation.

Recommended Dosage

IPAMORELIN RECOMMENDED DOSAGE

200-300 mcg injected subcutaneously one to three times a day.

It is recommended to cycle Ipamorelin for no longer than 8 weeks with an equal amount of time off for maximum efficacy.

Epitalon

Epitalon[77] is a derivative of Epithalamin, a naturally produced peptide found in your pineal gland.

It was discovered in the 1980s by Russian scientists and popularized by Dr. Vladmir Khavinson as a "bioregulator" to possibly prevent premature aging in Russia's military men.

Epitalon primarily works by increasing production of an enzyme called telomerase.

---

[77] http://pepbk.co/Epitalon

Telomerase allows our cells to produce protective parts of our DNA called telomeres.

Telomeres allow DNA to replicate and lead to the production of new cells.

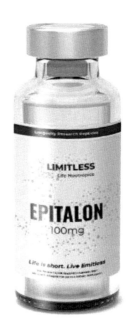

Our body's production of telomerase decreases over time.

This results in shorter telomeres which ultimately shortens our lifespan.

Consequently, our cells are eventually unable to divide or replicate, which leads to death of the physical body.

The more efficient our telomerase production as we age, the longer our telomeres extending our lifespan will be.

This provides our cells with a much lower biological age[78].

In several human studies conducted by Russian researchers, Epitalon supplementation led to lower mortality rates amongst the elderly and frail.

But even in healthy people, Epitalon can be used to improve sleep quality by increasing the body's natural production of the hormone melatonin.

Other possible benefits include better cardiovascular health, improved carbohydrate metabolism, and lowering age-associated impairment of physical endurance.

If your goal is **living a much longer life,** Epitalon is a must use anti-aging peptide.

Recommended Dosage

Just like MOTS-C, there doesn't appear to be a universal consensus on the dosing regimen for Epitalon.

There are several notable options to choose from.

---

[78] http://pepbk.co/BiologicalAge

EPITALON RECOMMENDED DOSAGE

• *The Khavinson Protocol*, according to Ben Greenfield: 10 mg of Epitalon injected subcutaneously three times a week for three weeks straight, done once a year.

• *An alternative Russian Protocol*, according to Dr. William Seeds in his book **Peptide Protocols, Volume 1**[79]: 10 mg of Epitalon injected intramuscularly every day for 10 days, done once every year for a total of two years.

• *The Ukrainian Protocol,* according to the International Peptide Society: 10 mg of Epitalon injected intramuscularly every THIRD day until you reach 50 mg total, done once every six months for a total of three years.

• *Dr. Heather Smith-Fernandez's protocol*: 1 mg of Epitalon injected subcutaneously every night.

---

[79] http://pepbk.co/PeptideProtocolsVol1

IMPORTANT NOTE

Epitalon MUST be administered via injection.

Any oral formulation would break the peptide down in the digestive tract and prevent it from entering the bloodstream.

In truth, most peptides only work if injected for the very same reasons.

If your physician is selling you tried and true injectable peptides as 'oral formulations', FIND ANOTHER ONE.

People often debate the best time to dose Epitalon.

Some users insist on injecting before bed to improve sleep.

Other users swear on a morning injection for more energy throughout the day.

Either way, Epitalon is best administered twice a year to stop cellular senescence[80] and to assist DNA repair through the upregulation of antioxidant production.

Due to its long-term anti-aging effects, be ready for the possibility you won't "notice" anything when

---

[80] http://pepbk.co/SenescentCells

administering Epitalon.

It's one of those unique peptides where a very short protocol "takes care of the results" for a very long period.

Epitalon can be used intermittently alongside other scheduled peptide therapies, so don't feel you have to stop using any of the peptides discussed in this book.

Thymalin

Thymalin[81] is a peptide spanning nine amino acids that is naturally produced in the thymus gland.

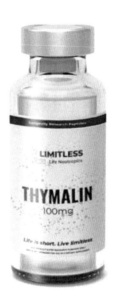

Thymalin was discovered in the 1970s by a French scientist.

However, it was Russian scientists in the 1980s that used Thymalin as a bioregulator to restore size and function to the thymus gland in aging men and women.

The thymus gland is responsible for regulating the body's immunity by allowing it to differentiate between naturally produced compounds and foreign substances entering the body.

---

[81] http://pepbk.co/Thymalin

Because the thymus gland "ages" faster than most organs in the body, it gradually decreases in size, minimizing its ability to maintain a robust immune system.

And thymalin production, like most naturally occurring peptides, also lowers with age.

Thymalin primarily works through *"T-cell differentiation and enhancement of T and NK cell actions"* (Wikipedia).

These are both key parts of the body's immune response.

While the role of this peptide as an immunity booster is crystal clear, the Russians also discovered Thymalin extends lifespan similarly to Epitalon.

When both peptides are used together, a much lower mortality rate is observed compared to using either peptide in isolation.

Other benefits observed include lower incidences of respiratory and cardiovascular disease, enhanced anti-inflammatory properties, and potential anti-tumor activity.

Thymalin is an excellent peptide for keeping the immune system fully functional as one ages.

For ultimate life extension purposes, you'll want to use

it in combination with Epitalon.

Recommended Dosage

 THYMALIN RECOMMENDED DOSAGE

Treating Immunity Disorders in Adults: **5-20 mg per day (30-100 mg total per course)**

Anti-Aging and Disease Prevention - **5-10 mg per day for adults**

Epitalon and Thymalin together are often a very synergistic combination - 5 mg EACH of Thymalin and Epitalon injected intramuscularly or subcutaneously once per day for 20 days straight, repeating every 6 months.

CHAPTER 5
THE BEST PEPTIDES FOR BRAIN FUNCTION AND COGNITIVE ENHANCEMENT

If you asked me about the best peptide for brain enhancement, I would say it depends on your goals.

Fortunately, there are enough peptides engineered or naturally produced to handle different aspects of brain health.

One may be the right choice for getting a competitive edge in the workplace, while another is better suited for the aging athlete focused on preventing neurological disease.

I've already written about these cognitive peptides in detail on my website[82].

As you've likely already gathered, the purpose of this book is providing you high-level summaries.

---

[82] http://pepbk.co/CognitivePeptides

IMPORTANT NOTE

Each peptide covered in this book includes a hyperlink to the full article on my website investigating all the technical details.

All linked articles are free and publicly available to read (provided you are signed up to my **email newsletter**[83]).

Semax

Semax[84] is a heptapeptide developed in Russia in the 1970s.

It is derived from a naturally produced hormone called "adrenocorticotropic hormone" (ACTH).

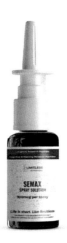

Human trials showed ACTH positively affected cognition but was unsuitable as a drug due to instability.

It's not FDA-approved, but Russia's own pharmaceutical regulatory agency approved the use of Semax in 1996

---

[83] http://pepbk.co/Newsletter
[84] http://pepbk.co/Semax

for multiple conditions.

Some of its most prominent uses include:

- *Reducing pain via the reduced breakdown of enkephalins, endogenous compounds known for lowering inflammation[85]*

- *Treating ischemic strokes*

- *Reversing undesirable effects of alcohol consumption via restoring function to the central nervous system*

- *Addressing the issues of various eye disorders*

- *Significantly improving memory and attention, even under extreme duress*

- *Increasing learning capacity and verbal fluency, likely through increased BDNF production.*

Overall, Semax is the most well rounded among the nootropic peptides.

It's neurorestorative, neuroprotective, and it provides a noticeable boost in cognition desired by most biohackers.

Where Semax really shines is when varying the dosages.

---

[85] http://pepbk.co/InflammatoryMarkers

While lower doses of Semax provide a boost in intellectual capacity, higher doses are used to address more serious conditions.

Semax is a preferred peptide for cognitive impairment when one is attempting to recover from a stroke.

It's no wonder researchers from the Russian Academy of Sciences coined Semax as "a universal drug for therapy and research" way back in 2008!

Recommended Dosage

The recommended doses for Semax are all over the place.

Here are the protocols I recommend that demonstrate the peptide's nootropic effects:

SEMAX RECOMMENDED DOSAGE

- **Dr. William Seeds, *Peptide Protocols* Vol. 1**[86]: 750-1000 mcg once a day if taken intranasally, 100-300 mcg once a day if injected subcutaneously.

- **Ben Greenfield in his book *Boundless***[87]: 0.5-1.0 mg per day when taken nasally or through subcutaneous injection.

- **Nick Andrews, world renowned formulator and co-creator of *The Peptides Course***[88]: 1.0-1.5 mg via intranasal spray when working very late nights due to Semax "providing a smooth burst of focus defeating fatigue without increasing alertness like caffeine".

Let's quickly do the math for the intranasal spray:

If your bottle contains 30 mg of Semax in a 10 mL

---

[86] http://pepbk.co/PeptideProtocolsVol1
[87] http://pepbk.co/Boundless
[88] http://pepbk.co/ThePeptidesCourse

solution, and each spray contains around 0.1-0.13 mL of solution, you're looking at 300 mcg of Semax per spray (i.e., 1-2 sprays in each nostril).

It's imperative you choose *either* the subcutaneous injection or the nasal spray for highest absorption rate.

Several studies have confirmed intranasal application to be the optimal route for experiencing the most pronounced cognitive enhancement.

Semax appears to be best taken in the morning fasted for maximum absorption via crossing the blood brain barrier.

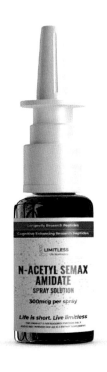

 IMPORTANT NOTE

You will hear the term "blood brain barrier" throughout this book when discussing the usage of therapeutic peptides.

The blood brain barrier is the barrier between the cerebral capillary blood and the interstitial fluid of the brain.

It is made up of capillary endothelial cells and functions primarily to prevent harmful substances from reaching the brain.

Peptides and many nutritional supplements function optimally when they are allowed to cross the blood brain barrier quickly and efficiently (in the absence of insulin (i.e., blood glucose) which competes with the agent for absorption).

This ensures maximum absorption and efficacy of the respective peptide and is best observed when a person is fasted.

You do not want Semax dosing to interfere with your sleep schedule.

(Many users have claimed testing nootropics at 3pm in the afternoon during an "energy lull" is the best way to confirm their energizing effects).

Note that the dosing recommendations I have provided are entirely different from the ones you would use for treating a brain stroke with Semax.

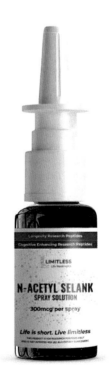

> ### ⚠ IMPORTANT NOTE
>
> **Christopher Mercer**[89], owner of Limitless Life Nootropics, prefers *n-acetyl semax amidate* over all other forms of Semax.
>
> This is due to its ability to better cross the blood brain barrier and extended half-life which leads to maximum absorption and efficacy.

Selank

Selank[90] is a synthetic analog of tuftsin, an immunomodulatory peptide found in humans.

As a heptapeptide (i.e., seven amino acids long), it stands out from many other peptides in that it serves two primary functions.

The primary purpose of Selank is to reduce anxiety.

---

[89] support@limitlesslifenootropics.com
[90] http://pepbk.co/Selank

Numerous human trials show it performs far better than drugs like benzodiazepines (which are highly addictive) and without the harmful side effects.

This is made possible through some of the same mechanisms responsible for Semax's nootropic properties:

- *Decreasing the rate at which enkephalins are degraded, which consequently decreases the anxiety response in humans*

- *Increasing BDNF production*

- *Lowering production of pro-inflammatory compounds in the brain*

- *Regulating the expression of dopamine and serotonin*

The secondary purpose of Selank is to provide boosts in learning speed and memory (both long and short-term).

These effects have only been confirmed by rat studies and the anonymous testimonials of brave biohackers.

So, while you can use Selank to give yourself a transient increase in brainpower, it's best to use it for calming yourself down and managing anxiety-associated conditions such as PTSD and ADHD.

Selank is clearly a much better treatment option than a

long course of antidepressants, stimulants, and tranquilizers that sick care medicine would prefer to supply you!

Recommended Dosage

The only reliable source for dosing Selank comes from notable peptide physician Dr. William Seeds, who recommends two separate routes in his book "**Peptide Protocols, Volume 1**"[91]:

SELANK RECOMMENDED DOSAGE

Subcutaneous Injection: 100-300 mcg of Selank once a day.

Intranasally (via nose spray): 750-1,000 mcg once a day, spread out over several doses if needed.

Some users report experiencing the anti-anxiety effects of Selank using as little as 250 mcg[92] administered intranasally.

Your results will vary due to the biochemical uniqueness of the end user.

---

[91] http://pepbk.co/PeptideProtocolsVol1
[92] http://pepbk.co/SelankReview

I personally would not go beyond Dr. Seeds' recommendations as it is possible to experience receptor attenuation (i.e., the target tissue becomes desensitized to Selank's effects).

As always, find the minimum effective dose needed to achieve satisfactory results and then slowly titrate the dosage when necessary.

When I spoke to Christopher Mercer, the owner of **Limitless Life Nootropics**[93], he gave me the following advice on finding the right dose of Selank:

> *"If you have a nasal spray bottle containing 30 mg of Selank, it will contain around 100 sprays (or 300 mcg per spray).*
>
> *Like Jay always says, start low and go slow from there.*
>
> *Selank is extremely safe and virtually impossible to overdose.*
>
> *You should notice the effects within 20 minutes of administration as they normally last for around 12 hours.*
>
> *In my view, the effects become more pronounced with each passing day"*

---

[93] http://pepbk.co/LimitlessLifeNootropics

If I had to choose either dosing option, I would go with the intranasal route.

Intranasal dosing appears to be the dosing strategy heavily suggested by the scientists at the Institute for Molecular Genetics of the Russian Academy of Sciences for the following reasons:

- *Rapid penetration through the blood brain barrier (so, lower doses may be administered)*

- *High bioavailability (92.8% of active ingredient)*

- *Fast clinical effect (the drug is detected in plasma and brain tissues in 30 sec and 2 min after administration)*

- *Concentration in archeocortex and interbrain (i.e., where Selank targets)*

- *Long-term action between 20 to 24 hours*

And long as you're going to be spraying your nostrils, this Reddit guide[94] is a great primer on how to properly use a nasal spray and store your Selank solution.

---

[94] http://pepbk.co/GuideToSemaxAndSelank

> ### ⚠ IMPORTANT NOTE
>
> **Christopher Mercer**[95], owner of Limitless Life Nootropics, prefers *n-acetyl selank amidate* over all other forms of Selank.
>
> This is due to its ability to better cross the blood brain barrier and extended half-life which leads to maximum absorption and efficacy.

Dihexa

Dihexa[96] is a six-amino-acid long peptide directly derived from Angiotensin IV (Ang IV), a metabolite of angiotensin II (a vasoconstrictor, i.e., increases blood pressure).

Like the discovery story of Semax, Angiotensin IV can enhance the acquisition and recall of information.

But because it is easily degraded, Angiotensin IV is unsuitable as a drug.

Thanks to the investigation of scientists into the structural properties of Angiotensin IV, it was

---

[95] support@limitlesslifenootropics.com
[96] http://pepbk.co/Dihexa

determined it had a specific structural motif responsible for its cognition-improving properties.

This structural motif was the basis for the creation of the nootropic peptide Dihexa.

And while we haven't seen human trials come to fruition, here's what we know about Dihexa so far:

- *It is orders of magnitude more powerful than BDNF in creating new neuronal connections and synapse formation*

- *Dihexa repairs already-occurred brain damage within the synapse between two nerve cells, rather than merely slow down the rate of disease progression in Alzheimer's (thus showing superior potential over existing treatments)*

Additionally, anecdotal reports from experimental human use claim Dihexa can shorten reaction time, boost mental endurance and improve one's problem-solving skills.

Much like Selank, I can't recommend using Dihexa as a nootropic.

I've personally used the peptide orally at varying dosages and it didn't do much with respect to cognitive enhancement.

Dihexa is the peptide you should pick if cognitive repair (in advance of a disease or during it) is your primary goal.

Recommended Dosage

DIHEXA RECOMMENDED DOSAGE

If you're looking for the right dosage of Dihexa for best results, the recommendations on the Internet vary significantly.

According to most anecdotal testimonials I've reviewed, the best Dihexa dose ranges anywhere between 8 mg and 45 mg taken daily.

The most popular method of administration is via transdermal application.

Typically, it is recommended to apply Dihexa cream onto the inner forearms until the cream is completely absorbed.

Other dosing methods have been utilized in examining the limited scientific evidence available for Dihexa.

The mice studies typically used an intravenous injection, while the ATH-1017 analog (a compound that supposedly gets converted into Dihexa in the body[97]) employs a once-a-day subcutaneous injection.

As I just mentioned earlier, I've only used Dihexa for a very short period and my results were mixed.

Because of this, I can't comment on what an optimal dosing protocol for Dihexa would be.

It is up to the reader to experiment with different doses and different modes of administration to see what works best for them.

Cerebrolysin

Cerebrolysin[98] is unlike other nootropic peptides in that it isn't a single peptide.

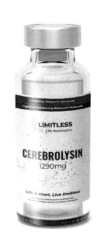

It is a complex mix of amino acids derived from pig brains and neuropeptides such as BDNF and nerve growth factor (NGF).

Cerebrolysin works primarily by stimulating protein synthesis and neuron growth.

---

[97] http://pepbk.co/NDX-1017vsDihexa
[98] http://pepbk.co/Cerebrolysin

In plain English: Cerebrolysin restores damaged neurons while protecting them from the onset of unwanted symptoms.

Since its discovery in 1949, there have been multiple tested applications of this peptide mixture in humans and animals.

Cerebrolysin has been shown to offer:

- *Better clinical outcomes in patients suffering from traumatic brain injury (TBI)*

- *Marked improvement in cognitive function within patients suffering from dementia*

- *Enhanced cognitive control in young adults with ADHD*

- *Potential promise in treating Alzhemier's disease regardless of whether high or low doses are used*

- *Improved mental function in children diagnosed with Autism/Asperger's*

The last one really caught my attention, especially when I saw the NIH (National Institutes of Health) publish this 2017 clinical trial from Russia[99]:

> *"Forty-three children with autism spectrum*

---

[99] http://pepbk.co/CerebrolysinAutism

disorders, aged 4-6 years, were included in the study.

To assess the degree of autism, the quantitative scale of assessing the severity of child autism CARS ('Childhood Autism Rating Scale') was used. "

"In children with exogenous (organic) autism, the lower scores of autistic symptoms on the CARS and a greater degree of functional immaturity of the cerebral cortex, according to electroencephalographic results, were found compared to children with endogenous autism.

After treatment with Cerebrolysin, 27 children (62.8%) showed signs of improvement.

An improvement was noted in 13 children with endogenous autism (56.5%) and in 14 children with organic autism (70.0%).

CARS scores showed a more pronounced decrease in this indicator in a subgroup of children with organic autism."

While its primary use is best suited for preventing memory loss and cognitive decline, healthy people can also use it to improve memory and cognitive functioning.

Think of Cerebrolysin as more of a "neuroprotective" peptide for optimal brain health, rather than a focusing agent like Modafinil[100] for enhanced focus and or wakefulness.

As for the Russian autism study, larger trials run on North American soil would be optimal to potentially observe Cerebrolysin as a viable treatment option for various levels of autism.

Recommended Dosage

If you look online for the best dose of Cerebrolysin to get the highest levels of neuroprotection possible, you'll find most dosing schemes are designed for people suffering from neurodegeneration:

---

[100] http://pepbk.co/Modafinil

CEREBROLYSIN RECOMMENDED DOSAGE

Disorder	Daily Dosage	Duration of treatment
Stroke	20 - 50 ml	10 - 21 days
Traumatic Brain Injury	20 - 50 ml	7 - 30 days
Vascular Dementia	20 - 50 ml	1 cycle: 5 days weekly/4 weeks 2 - 4 cycles per year
Alzheimer's Disease	20 - 50 ml	1 cycle: 5 days weekly/4 weeks 2 - 4 cycles per year

Initiation of treatment for all disorders should be **as soon as possible**

Source: **http://pepbk.co/HowToUseCerebrolysin**

The official website for Cerebrolysin recommends keeping the peptide stored in a dry place at room temperature and removed from exposure to direct sunlight.

These recommendations are based on the version of

Cerebrolysin consisting of "*active substance cerebrolysin concentrate (complex of peptides obtained from the porcine brain tissue), 215.2 mg per 1 mL.*"

As for the best Cerebrolysin dosage to take for enhanced cognition in healthy adults:

The overall consensus seems to be 5-10 mL injected subcutaneously once a day for a single cycle of 10-20 days.

Even then, there are some disagreements amongst biohackers regarding the best dosing protocol for Cerebrolysin.

While some people cycle Cerebrolysin on and off for maximum effect, others claim cycling Cerebrolysin is not necessary and can be used consistently when needed.

You will also see claims that intramuscular injections (and intravenous injections in some cases) are more effective than subcutaneous injections, although this is entirely subjective to the end user.

As with nearly all the peptides endorsed in this book, one must experiment with Cerebrolysin to see which dosage, frequency and method of administration works best.

Orexin A

Orexin A[101] is a 33-amino-acid peptide that is predominantly located in the hypothalamus region of the brain.

It is part of a family of neuropeptides known as "orexins", which are integral for cognitive health[102]:

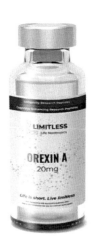

> *"The Orexin/Orexin Receptor (OXR) system plays a vital role in multiple functions of the central nervous system (CNS), including modulation of the sleep— wake rhythm cycle, reward systems feeding behavior, energy homeostasis, and cardiovascular responses, as well as cognition and mood.*
>
> *...Dysfunction of the orexin system has been implicated in many pathological conditions, including narcolepsy, insomnia, depression, ischemic stroke, addiction, and Alzheimer's disease (AD)"*
>
> *- Krithika Subramanian, PhD*

While it was initially discovered as a peptide that increases feeding behavior, scientists accidentally found Orexin A played a large role in wakefulness.

---

[101] http://pepbk.co/Orexin-A
[102] http://pepbk.co/Orexins

(NOTE: Obviously, Orexin A is not a peptide to use when attempting to lose body fat. But it is a great companion when one is attempting to gain lean muscle mass yet struggles to consume enough calories.)

When the body is deficient in Orexin A (i.e., low in neurons responsible for producing it), one isn't aroused while awake and far more likely to return to sleep for long periods of time.

For this reason, Orexin A is used as a treatment for narcolepsy when cataplexy is present (i.e., sudden muscle weakness while you are fully alert).

From the few testimonials of Orexin A I could find online, many people claim Orexin A's wakefulness-enhancing properties allowed them to stay energized while eliminating their reliance on ADHD medication.

It's quite like Modafinil: Orexin A doesn't so much enhance cognition as it puts one in a state where they retain wakefulness for longer periods of time.

This offsets the cognitive decline associated with a lack of polyphasic (i.e., deep restorative) sleep.

I can't say for sure if it's going to replace Modafinil, but Orexin A is worth looking into if you're seeking an alternative.

Recommended Dosage

Based on the compilation of biohackers' experiences (truly the only data we have in helping healthy people enhance daytime alertness), the following protocol seems optimal:

OREXIN A RECOMMENDED DOSAGE

The best Orexin A dosage would be 100-150 mcg administered intranasally once a day in the early morning.

Although I was able to find one instance of users dosing 250mcg via intramuscular injection once per day, it is important to note they were using it alongside peptides such as Ipamorelin, CJC-1295, and P21[103].

If you're unsure of how you'll react to Orexin A on your first dose, start low with 50 mcg and gradually titrate your dosage upward.

---

[103] http://pepbk.co/P21

FGL

FGL (a.k.a. the Fibroblast Growth Loop peptide)[104] is a 15-amino-acid long peptide that supports the growth and development of neurons, hence why it is known as a "neurotrophic" peptide.

There are numerous mechanisms through which FGL purportedly helps people learn and retain new information.

None of these mechanisms appear to be more significant than one another with respect to available data.

We also have mechanistic studies in cell cultures and rats that show promise in the following areas:

- *Protecting against neurotoxicity*

- *Possessing anti-neuroinflammatory properties*

- *Promoting neuron survival and synapse formation*

- *Possible treatment of psychiatric disorders*

- *Promoting cognitive recovery after stroke and TBI*

Due to the lack of human trials, FGL is one of the more experimental nootropic peptides in the marketplace.

---

[104] http://pepbk.co/FGL

The biohacking community is also mixed on this peptide.

While many claim their brains have become more attuned to learning and maintaining a positive mood, Nick Andrews did not notice any significant effects after taking extremely high doses of FGL every day.

So, unlike the other peptides, I'm leaving the rest to you.

Experiment with it yourself and see if it boosts your brainpower in a meaningful way.

Recommended Dosage

 FGL RECOMMENDED DOSAGE

The optimal FGL dose is **1-2 mg injected subcutaneously** into your abdomen once per day on a "5 day on, 2 days off" cycle, according to Dr. William Seeds in his book **Peptide Protocols, Volume 1**[105].

He advises younger individuals in their thirties and under to stick with 1 mg while following his protocol for six weeks to assess how you feel.

---

[105] http://pepbk.co/PeptideProtocolsVol1

PE-22-28

PE-22-28[106] was brought to my attention when I was looking for peptides that exclusively focus on mood regulation.

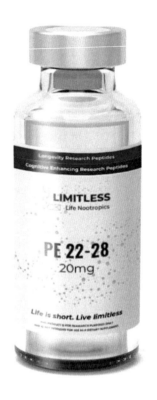

The only thing I can reliably say about PE-22-28 is that it is the "antidepressant" peptide among the peptides listed in this book.

This is based on numerous rat studies where the peptide was shown to lower the incidence of maladaptive depressive behaviors, especially in situations of chronically elevated stress.

But what makes it a standout candidate for treating depression is how it proved to be superior to antidepressants in the following ways:

- *Faster onset of action (days for PE-22-28 versus weeks for traditional antidepressants)*

- *No negative effects on sleep*

- *No observation of withdrawal symptoms*

---

[106] http://pepbk.co/PE-22-28

- *Absence of common side effects usually seen with antidepressants*

While its use is far more targeted than FGL, it also belongs in the class of highly experimental peptides lacking both empirical data (from end users) and meaningful clinical research.

Recommended Dosage

I defer to *Dr. Elizabeth Yurth* for her expertise since she's the ONLY physician I know who has direct experience with using PE-22-28 on patients suffering from major depressive disorders:

 PE-22-28 RECOMMENDED DOSAGE

The best PE-22-28 dosage for depression is 400 mcg administered intranasally once a day in the morning.

If you can obtain PE-22-28 from a source that requires reconstitution into a nasal spray, this video tutorial[107] is very helpful in understanding how to properly prepare it for administration.

---

[107] http://pepbk.co/DIYIntranasalPE-22-28

Melanotan I

Melanotan I[108] was saved for last because it doesn't really enhance cognition like the other nootropic peptides do.

Rather than help you memorize information or focus better, "M1" (as it's affectionately known) helps to increase consciousness.

And what could be better than that, my friends, to save this planet from impending destruction?

I'll quote myself from **Living A Fully Optimized Life**[109], where I talk about how Melanotan 1's melanin-increasing characteristic is the gateway to increasing consciousness, i.e. raising your vibration:

> *"[Melanin] can stimulate the pineal gland.*
>
> *The pineal gland secretes the hormone melatonin (primarily during the hours of 2 a.m. to 6 a.m.), which literally bathes the brain and creates the chemical condition necessary for "inner vision" to take place.*
>
> *It is Jay's awareness (based on empirical observation of his own life) that using [Melanotan I] has helped significantly in his spiritual evolution*

---

[108] http://pepbk.co/Melanotan1
[109] http://pepbk.co/LAFOL

and connection to "WHAT IS" (a.k.a. his inner knowing expressed as the higher SELF or the divine connection to one's holy spirit essence)."

It's not something I can easily describe, unlike my experiences with 5-MeO-DMT[110] and the RASHA Technology[111].

I recommend reading those two articles if you want the best 3D description of what enhanced consciousness feels like.

And on a side note, it provides a more even skin tan compared to Melanotan II[112].

Recommended Dosage

The optimal dose of Melanotan I depends entirely on what you are using it for.

Listed are my own recommendations along with dosing strategies of other trusted experts.

---

[110] http://pepbk.co/5-MeO-DMT
[111] http://pepbk.co/RASHA
[112] http://pepbk.co/Melanotan2

MELATONAN 1 RECOMMENDED DOSAGE

Enhancing Consciousness: A minimum effective dose (MED) of 0.25 mg injected subcutaneously 1-2 times in the morning[113] per week.

I have been using Melanotan I on and off for close to 12 years.

I can confirm this is the appropriate dose to use year-round for maximizing conscious awareness while minimizing any potential side effects (there rarely are any).

MELATONAN 1 RECOMMENDED DOSAGE

Skin Tanning: 0.5 mg injected subcutaneously twice per day, increasing the daily dosage to 1.5 per mg by the third or fourth day and then stopping after one week.

I recommend doing this no more than 8 months out of the year.

---

[113] http://pepbk.co/SupplementProtocol

Sunlight exposure (i.e., UV-B exposure) while using Melanotan I is imperative if you want the fastest and longest-lasting results from tanning.

Alternatively, notable peptide physician Dr. William Seeds[114] recommends a subcutaneous injection of 200 mcg once per day for a week, adjusting the dose according to pigment changes.

He then recommends transitioning to 100 mcg twice a week after pigment stabilization.

And while I don't wholeheartedly believe in dosing based on your specific shade of skin color, this small guide[115] is helpful for those of you who insist on making this kind of adjustment.

MELATONAN 1 RECOMMENDED DOSAGE

Immunity: I personally do not use Melanotan I for this purpose, but Dr. Seeds[116] recommends 200 mcg injected subcutaneously once per day for 6-8 weeks until the clinical effects are more pronounced.

[114] http://pepbk.co/PeptideProtocolsVol1
[115] http://pepbk.co/Melanotan1Instructions
[116] http://pepbk.co/PeptideProtocolsVol1

Dr. Seeds claims Melanotan I is very effective for autoimmune conditions.

He also states a noticeably positive side effect of sexual stimulation is observed in some users (especially at higher doses of 500 – 1,000 mcg).

Melanotan I's use, as you can see, is very straightforward.

Positive results will come if anyone uses the peptide as recommended in this book.

CHAPTER 6
THE BEST PEPTIDES FOR ENHANCING IMMUNITY

The best peptides for your immune system aren't so much "boosters" as they are regulators of immunity.

In other words, peptides for immunity help maintain an optimal balance of immune cells[117] in the body (i.e., homeostasis) via the stimulation or suppression of the body's immune response.

Therefore, you'll often see peptides referred to as "immuno-modulating agents" when you look them up in the medical literature.

Many of these peptides are naturally found in your body and can be re-administered into your system exactly as they are if you know how to make them properly.

There are currently 3 peptides for immune system regulation I would recommend.

Fortunately, most of them either target immunity solely or have immune system modulation as one of their primary effects.

---

[117] http://pepbk.co/ImmuneSystemDisorders

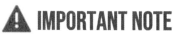

⚠ IMPORTANT NOTE

TB-500[118] and BPC-157[119] have already been heavily covered for their profound healing and regenerative effects on my website[120].

They both also offer an immune enhancing effect but it's not what they are primarily used for.

Because both BPC-157 and TB-500 are two of the most well known peptides to the casual observer, I AM covering them later in the bonus chapter:

How To Heal Like X-Men's Wolverine for the fastest injury repair and recovery possible.

Thymosin-Alpha 1

In the 2023 world of bioweapons, COVID and compromised health, what is the #1 therapeutic peptide to strengthen our immunity?

Thymosin Alpha-1[121] (better known by its users as TA-1) is an amazingly powerful peptide for strengthening the immune system and lowering your risk of infection (if not preventing it altogether).

---

[118] http://pepbk.co/TB-500
[119] http://pepbk.co/BPC-157
[120] http://pepbk.co/TB-500AndBPC-157
[121] http://pepbk.co/TA-1

TA-1 is a peptide that progressive health optimization doctors frequently use with their high-level clients because it demonstrates promise across multiple disease states[122].

It is truly profound in its efficacy and one of the peptides I recommend never leaving home without when traveling the globe.

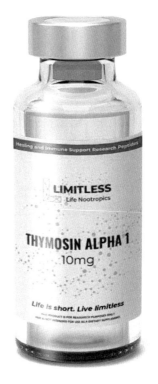

Thymosin Alpha-1 (TA-1) is a 28-amino-acid peptide naturally produced in the thymus gland, which itself is responsible for regulating the immune system.

Thymosin-Alpha-1 is what "signals" the T-cells to be released from the thymus gland.

In terms of the peptide's history, it was first discovered by scientist Allan L. Goldstein and his colleagues in 1977 when they wanted to determine if the thymus gland's immune-boosting effects were hormonal in nature.

After isolating a group of small proteins known as "thymosins" from the calf tissue of cows, further

122 http://pepbk.co/TA-1Wiki

purification and isolation of these compounds led to the identification of an active component known as "Thymosin Fraction 5" (TF5).

And following some positive results with using TF5 in humans and animals suffering from a variety of immunity-related diseases, they wanted to see if a SPECIFIC part of TF5 was responsible for its effects.

This led to the eventual isolation and characterization of Thymosin Alpha-1[123].

TA-1 is so powerful it enhances immunity in people with severely compromised thymus glands[124] (or none at all according to experimental animal studies).

Goldstein himself even said[125] that Thymosin Alpha-1 is *"10-1000 times more active than fraction 5 in several assay systems in vitro and in vivo designed to measure T cell differentiation and function."*

Several decades later, we now know that Thymosin Alpha-1 does wonders for enhancing the strength of your immune system.

Thymosin Alpha-1 is regarded as an incredibly strong immunomodulator.

---

[123] http://pepbk.co/TA-1Isolation
[124] http://pepbk.co/TA-1Immunodeficiency
[125] http://pepbk.co/TA-1Goldstein

The Merriam-Webster Dictionary defines this as "*a chemical agent that modifies the immune response or the functioning of the immune system (as by the stimulation of antibody formation or the inhibition of white blood cell activity)*".

 IMPORTANT NOTE

Thymosin Alpha-1 is one of the FEW FDA-Approved peptides in existence.

Many of the peptides I write about (and mentioned in this book) have yet to be approved by the Food and Drug Administration (FDA) for select medical purposes.

All peptide drugs currently approved by the United States Food and Drug Association (FDA) are found in this online table[126].

All peptide drugs currently undergoing clinical trials as of 2022 are found in this online table[127].

Thymosin Alpha-1 is an FDA-approved prescription drug known as Zadaxin (thymalfasin) manufactured by SciClone Pharmaceuticals.

Without diving into the details, TA-1 currently has the

[126] http://pepbk.co/FDAApprovedPeptides
[127] http://pepbk.co/PeptidesInClinicalTrials

status of an Orphan Drug[128] designated to treat malignant melanoma, Hepatitis B, and hepatocellular carcinoma (i.e., liver cancer).

How does Thymosin Alpha-1 work, you may ask?

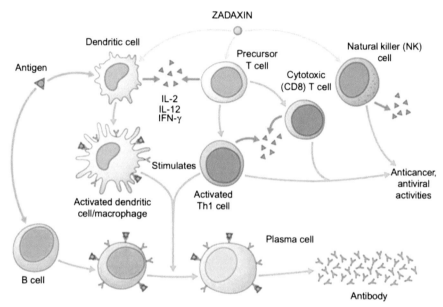

Image Source[129]

One of Thymosin Alpha-1's primary mechanisms involve stimulating the production of cytotoxic T-cells[130].

Thymosin Alpha-1 also activates natural killer (NK) cells[131], which are responsible for mediating the immune system's response against tumors and viruses.

[128] http://pepbk.co/Thymalfasin
[129] http://pepbk.co/TA-1ImmuneModulation
[130] http://pepbk.co/TA-1THPdb
[131] http://pepbk.co/TA-1NKCells

Additionally, Thymosin Alpha-1 is responsible for the maturation and differentiation of dendritic cells[132] (which are antigen-presenting cells responsible for activating the adaptive immune system):

As I wrote previously when discussing the peptide Thymalin[133], the primary reason our immunity tends to weaken with age is due to the shrinking of the thymus gland[134] and its consequent loss of optimal function.

Here is a list of the potential disease states and negative reactions from the body not producing enough Thymosin Alpha-1 as one ages:

- *Chronic fatigue, physical exhaustion, tired appearance, lack of motivation, apathy, chronic infections (colds, herpes, hepatitis, shingles, lyme, and other severe infections)*

- *Persistent illness, lack of full recovery, e.g., recurrent bouts of "flu-like" symptoms, CFIDS (Chronic Fatigue Immune Dysfunction Syndrome)*

- *Easily injured joints, ligaments, tendons, and muscles with slow recovery*

- *Chronic pain and disability after musculoskeletal trauma*

---

[132] http://pepbk.co/TA-1DendriticCells
[133] http://pepbk.co/Thymalin
[134] http://pepbk.co/ThymicInvolution

- *Slow, difficult, and incomplete wound healing*

Chronically low Thymosin Alpha-1 levels is one of the surest signs immunity has been compromised[135].

Put another way, immune-compromised individuals – especially those suffering from chronic inflammatory autoimmune diseases (about as run of the mill as anything in adults who suffer from "Long COVID") – have far lower levels of Thymosin Alpha-1[136] compared to healthy adults.

As if you needed any more reason to make TA-1 a staple in your peptide arsenal, here are the 7 primary health benefits it provides according to the clinical literature:

- *Effective against common flus and colds*

- *Enhances the effect of cancer treatments*

- *May help treat hepatitis B & C*

- *Shows great potential for treating HIV-1*

- *Improves rate of recovery from sepsis*

- *Massively suppresses chronic inflammation*

- *May lower chronic fatigue*

---

[135] http://pepbk.co/TA-1Levels
[136] http://pepbk.co/TA-1ChronicDisease

Recommended Dosage

The most optimal dosing protocol for Thymosin Alpha-1 is relatively straightforward[137]:

 THYMOSIN-ALPHA 1 RECOMMENDED DOSAGE

1.5 mg of Thymosin Alpha-1 injected subcutaneously (i.e., in your belly fat) twice a week in evenly spaced doses.

Doses of 1.0-1.5 mg taken twice a week are also observed in clinical trials[138] involving hepatitis B/C and HIV/AIDS, so don't worry about adjusting this dose for a human being.

You can take as much as 1.5 mg of Thymosin Alpha-1 per day, or even use micro doses on a "5 day on, 2 days off" protocol.

If it's not obvious by now, TA-1 is an incredibly potent peptide, and you only need minute amounts to experience a profound effect.

Keep in mind that Thymosin Alpha-1 reaches peak

---

[137] http://pepbk.co/TA-1Protocol
[138] http://pepbk.co/TA-1HIVAIDS

concentration in your body around ~80 minutes after the injection[139] and has a half-life of 2 hours, which means it acts very rapidly.

The next two immunity enhancing peptides are also great, but not as clinically well understood as TA-1.

Because we are unable to "trust the science" as deeply as we'd like on TA-1, I AM only covering them as high-level summaries.

Deeper dives on each are found in their respective articles on my website.

LL-37

LL-37[140] is a peptide spanning 37 amino acids that is directly derived from an antimicrobial peptide called "cathelicidin."

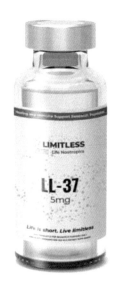

A cathelicidin is a *"cationic antimicrobial peptide (AMP) in which a highly conserved N-terminal structural domain, cathelin, is linked to a C-terminal peptide with antimicrobial activity"* (Source[141]).

[139] http://pepbk.co/TA-1Concentration
[140] http://pepbk.co/LL-37
[141] http://pepbk.co/Cathelicidin

To be more exact, LL-37 is derived from the region of the only known human cathelicidin to exist (a.k.a. hCAP18) that has antimicrobial properties.

This peptide works mostly through binding to the pathogen's cellular membrane and leaking out the contents within the pathogen's cell, ultimately leading to cellular death.

The benefits of LL-37 can be summed in three words:

1. *Anti-bacterial*

2. *Anti-fungal*

3. *Anti-viral*

LL-37 has often been lauded as a possibly superior treatment option compared to antibiotics based on its broad-spectrum activity and lower levels of treatment resistance without harming the host organism.

However, the COVID-19 pandemic saw LL-37 re-emerge as a possibly effective therapeutic:

> *"SARS-CoV-2 infection begins with the association of its spike 1 (S1) protein with host angiotensin-converting enzyme-2 (ACE2).*
>
> *Targeting the interaction between S1 and ACE2 is a practical strategy against SARS-CoV-2 infection.*

Herein, we show encouraging results indicating that human cathelicidin LL37 can simultaneously block viral S1 and cloak ACE2"(Source[142])

"We hypothesize upregulation of LL-37 will act therapeutically, facilitating efficient NET clearance by macrophages, speeding endothelial repair after inflammatory tissue damage, preventing α-synuclein aggregation, and supporting blood-glucose level stabilization by facilitating insulin release and islet β-cell neogenesis.

In addition, it has been postulated that LL-37 can directly bind the S1 domain of SARS-CoV-2, mask angiotensin converting enzyme 2 (ACE2) receptors, and limit SARS-CoV-2 infection. "(Source[143])

Making a much longer story short: LL-37 can be considered your go-to anti-bacterial and/or anti-viral peptide, especially in the very early days of infection.

Recommended Dosage

The dosage recommendations for LL-37 seem to differ depending on who you ask, but they all fit within a tight range.

---

[142] http://pepbk.co/CathelicidinInhibitsCOVID
[143] http://pepbk.co/CathelicidinSevereCOVID

LL-37 RECOMMENDED DOSAGE

Carl Lanore of SuperHuman Radio[144] recommends 125 mcg per day injected subcutaneously for 50 days, followed by a 2-4 week break before doing a second round if necessary.

Dr. William Seeds[145] recommends 100 mcg of LL-37 injected subcutaneously twice a day (once in morning and once at night) for 4-6 weeks.

As I always say, you and you alone are 100% responsible for how you use this peptide and how you react to it.

Start with the minimum effective dose possible (starting low and going slow), monitor your body's reactions, and use common sense.

VIP

Vasoactive intestinal peptide (VIP)[146] was initially discovered in the 1960s as a vasodilator that is produced in numerous parts of the human body.

---

[144] http://pepbk.co/LL-37SuperHumanRadio
[145] http://pepbk.co/LL-37Seeds
[146] http://pepbk.co/VIPeptide

Indeed, it is very good at reducing high blood pressure, improving oxygenation[147] (i.e., getting oxygen from the lungs and pushing it throughout the body), and relaxing the larger airway passages within the lungs.

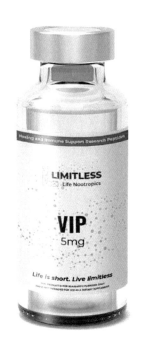

But within its long laundry list of health benefits, you'll also find its simultaneous involvement in both innate and adaptive immunity.

So, on top of activating the cells needed to prevent pathogen movement within the body, it can also activate the cells needed to generate immunity to a specific pathogen.

And when it comes to COVID-19, more VIP production reduces your chances of suffering from severe illness[148]:

> *"...plasma levels of the immunoregulatory neuropeptide VIP are elevated in patients with severe COVID-19, correlating with reduced inflammatory mediators and with survival on those patients.*

---

[147] http://pepbk.co/VIPOxygenation
[148] http://pepbk.co/VIPCOVID

In vitro, vasoactive intestinal peptide (VIP) and pituitary adenylate cyclase-activating polypeptide (PACAP), highly similar neuropeptides, decreased the SARS-CoV-2 RNA content in human monocytes and viral production in lung epithelial cells, also reducing cell death."

And especially for COVID-19 patients suffering from severe comorbidities, VIP can be used as a treatment to increase survivability and recover fully from respiratory failure.

Put another way: If VIP production is blocked by COVID-19, you will find yourself unable to breathe and needing a ventilator (effectively a death sentence).

VIP is recommended for general immunity but is especially useful as the "magic bullet" against any illness involving respiratory problems and/or lack of good blood flow.

Recommended Dosage

Sadly, we do not have a universal dosing protocol in existence for VIP.

Combined with its limited use in humans and its extremely broad spectrum of biological effects, it's hard to give a blanket recommendation.

VIP RECOMMENDED DOSAGE

The standard protocol for administering VIP[149] seems to be 50 mcg sprayed intranasally within each nostril up to 4 times per day for a total of 30-90 days (with the goal of gradually reducing the dose to zero).

While some functional medicine physicians claim VIP can be used safely[150] alongside peptides such as BPC-157[151], I do not have the experience, nor do I know anybody who has tried this.

Biohackers claim better results with a subcutaneous injection[152] instead of an intranasal spray, but I also don't have the knowledge to confirm this.

Therefore, you are entirely on your own to experiment and determine how much VIP you should be using and how often to use it.

---

[149] http://pepbk.co/VIPProtocol
[150] http://pepbk.co/VIPAndBPC-157
[151] http://pepbk.co/BPC-157
[152] http://pepbk.co/VIPInjection

CHAPTER 7
THE BEST PEPTIDES FOR SKIN/HAIR CARE

No other peptide deserves to be positively recommended in this book more than copper peptide GHK-Cu[153].

It is truly the "sham wow" of peptides due to its multi-functional capabilities in cellular healing and regeneration.

It improves skin density and firmness while reducing fine lines and deep wrinkles.

It also dramatically improves skin clarity while helping to tighten loose skin.

Many of my friends have also noted its ability to treat sunburn, especially in fair complexioned people.

Copper peptide GHK-Cu is a topical solution that works systemically.

It can be topically applied to any part of the body and heal the specific site of the injury locally (no injections necessary).

Even better is that GHK-Cu combined with Carbon 60[154]

---

[153] http://pepbk.co/GHK-Cu
[154] http://pepbk.co/C60

(C60) helps to regrow hair.

Here's an email I received from a "Geoffrey" in 2020 where he told me how potent this combination is:

> *"Hey Jay!*
>
> *I heard you talk about a new product you're in process of making with GHK-Cu and Carbon 60.*
>
> *I've been using Tailor MADE GHK-Cu for about 6 months and have noticeably increased hair growth (see first pic).*
>
> *About two months ago, I started using C60 in combination with the GHK-Cu and I have been getting phenomenal results with these two combined.*
>
> *If you create an all-in-one hair topical, I believe you will make a massive impact on hair restoration.*
>
> *Check out my results."*

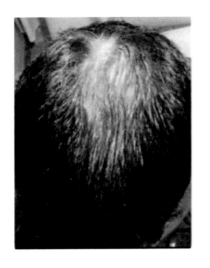 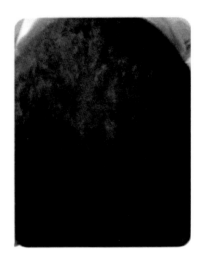

Before   **After**

As I mentioned in a previous chapter, reputable suppliers of GHK-Cu-based products are currently in short supply.

As high-quality ones become available, you may visit **pepbk.co/GHK-CuProducts** to view my most up-to-date recommendation(s).

⚠ IMPORTANT NOTE

Rules for Stacking Peptides.

It's important to understand that "stacking peptides" is relevant to your goal.

You can't stack a fat Loss peptide with a muscle gain peptide and expect to have the best results because your lifestyle (epigenetics) must be relevant to your primary goal.

Meaning if your primary goal is muscle gain, then you must increase calories (beyond maintenance intake) which would automatically prevent you (as the end user) from also losing body fat (where a caloric deficit over time is required).

As stated previously many times in this book already, peptides are not magic bullets.

One must prioritize a specific goal and focus on it over time rather than attempt to solve multiple issues with multiple peptides at the same time.

Here are some specific examples where stacking peptides is not counterproductive to the primary goal of the end user:

A Healing Stack[155] for an acute injury would be TB-500 and BPC-157.

A Fat Loss Stack[156] for a heavy-set person would be MOTS-C along with Ipamorelin or Tesamorelin.

An Immunity Stack[157] would be TA-1 used in precise micro-dose fashion during or in combo with a Fat Loss or Muscle Gain stack.

A Muscle Gain Stack[158] is Ipamorelin and Tesamorelin combined. Throw in 5-Amino 1MQ (if money is not an objection) for you.

A Cognition Enhancing Stack would be two of the Nootropic peptides used together.

I don't recommend stacking two neuro-enhancing peptides together and would prefer users choose one nootropic peptide that produces a noticeable effect and stay there.

---

[155] http://pepbk.co/WolverineHealingStack
[156] http://pepbk.co/FatLossStack
[157] http://pepbk.co/ImmuneBoostingPeptides
[158] http://pepbk.co/MuscleGrowthStack

CONCLUSION

First, congratulations on making it this far into the book.

The sad reality is that most people don't!

The information found in this book about peptides is dense.

It requires a certain amount of intelligence, patience, and discipline to get all the way through.

In my experience, most people simply don't want to DO THE WORK to educate themselves.

If you've been able to read, process, and digest this information, you are *well* ahead of most of the population (and even most doctors!).

Maybe you've arrived at this point and realize much of this information has literally gone over your head?

You may feel like you're in the dark regarding the science of peptides and unsure about the principles and recommendations we've touched on.

Wherever you find yourself is exactly where the universe wants you to be.

My advice is to go through this information as many

times as necessary to learn about the peptides that apply to you and your unique situation.

Don't hesitate to take notes and come back to certain concepts and ideas.

Because once you TRULY have a solid understanding of peptides, you'll be ready to move onto the fun part: **taking action.**

Having read up to this point, are you ready to start using peptides?

I have been using therapeutic peptides since 2004.

This was well before most in the medical community even knew what they were.

To say I have mastered their usage since then would be an understatement.

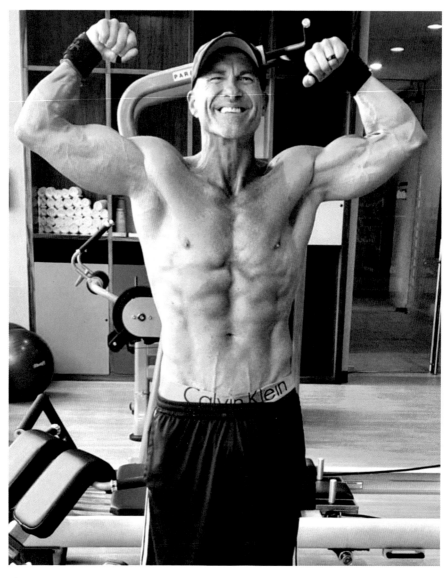

This is me at nearly 52 years young (August 2022).

I AM supremely confident I can help you optimize your physical body in the context of long-term health and safety when using therapeutic peptides to meet your goals.

I recently created a digital course that condenses my nearly two decades of experience into a step-by-step guide.

It will make you an expert using therapeutic peptides to radically optimize your health.

The **Therapeutic Peptides Course**[159] is designed for men and women who truly desire to be in the top 1% of humanity.

Men and women who are unwilling to wait for the "mainstream science" to catch up (it will be decades).

If you are ready for exponential growth at a body and soul level, my course is your ticket.

Keep reading to see all the content you'll get immediate access to when you purchase the course.

---

[159] http://pepbk.co/ThePeptidesCourse

TAKING THE NEXT STEP

The Therapeutic Peptides Course is THE biohacker's answer to using therapeutic peptides to burn fat, build muscle, heal injuries, reduce cognitive decline, improve health, and slow aging.

As a health-conscious individual who has likely listened to many of my podcasts and read my articles about peptides (and even this book), you may still be slightly unsure of what peptides to use, how to use them, or where to even find them.

That's quite alright.

My online course will be your step-by-step guide.

Along with my business partner and co-author Nick Andrews *(a biochemical engineer with 20+ years of extensive experience in the bio-pharma space and in formulating therapeutic peptides)*, we walk you all the way through the process to meet your desired outcome.

All you must do is watch, listen and learn.

When you purchase the course, you'll get access to the following six modules.

(For more information about The Therapeutic Peptides course, visit **pepbk.co/ThePeptidesCourse**)

And because you purchased this book, you'll receive a
special discount when you use the coupon code
PEPTIDESBOOK at checkout!

(Note: The Advanced version of the course contains multiple bonus lessons and special offers-well worth the price of entry if you're serious about peptides.)

Module 1: Understanding Regenerative Medicine: Utilizing Your Body's Systems for Self-Repair

Before we can begin any discussion of using therapeutic peptides for medical purposes, we'll revisit some basic high school biochemistry to understand our genetic code and the role peptides play in it.

Self-healing may seem like a superpower only seen in movies, but it's rooted in more reality than you might think.

When you get a cut, your body heals.

Your fingernail falls off, it grows back.

This happens on a cellular level, too, and in this module, we'll provide a high-level overview of your body's natural ability to self-repair and how peptides can aid it.

We'll dive into:

- *Understanding your genetic code (and how peptides are the key to unlocking it)*

- *The differences between allopathic (sick care or illness medicine) and regenerative medicine*

- *What you must understand about how large medical studies are conducted (and how to use the findings to assess your own personal risk)*

- *The pros, cons, and risks of using peptides*

We'll use the following tools:

- **A Guide to Understanding Regenerative Medicine** so you understand not just what, but why, and how

- **Glossary of Terms** so you always know what we're referring to throughout the program to get the most out of the course content

- **Risk Factors Cheat Sheet** so you can clearly see potential red flags

Module 2: Symptoms and Solutions: The 4 Classes of Peptides

Each of us naturally produce a wide variety of peptides throughout our lives as part of our bodies' normal healthy function and regulation.

As we age and expose ourselves to different diets (i.e., GMO-processed foods), physical and mental changes, and environmental stressors (i.e., endocrine-disrupting compounds), the production of these peptides gets down-regulated.

Over time, our ability to heal faster also slows down.

Utilizing therapeutic peptides unlocks your body's natural healing abilities.

In this module, we'll give you all the information you need to know about the **four classes of peptides** we're covering in the course:

- *Aesthetics (Body Composition Change) & Athletic Performance*

- *Healing/Injury Recovery*

- *Enhancing Immunity*

- *Increasing Mental Performance*

By the end of this module, you'll understand:

A. What peptides to use in order to achieve the results you want and
B. How they work.

We'll also dive into:

- *How peptides can help with both chronic and acute issues*

- *What peptides can help you start regenerating injured tissue and lowering healing time*

- *The most effective peptides for enhancing fat loss, building lean muscle, preventing depression, and improving overall wellbeing*

- *The best peptides to enhance immunity in the age of COVID (and what kind of results you can expect)*

- *The four best peptides for enhancing cognitive function (and what kind of results you can expect)*

We'll use the following tools:

- **Peptides Class Worksheets** so you understand how they work in your body and what to expect when using them

Module 3: Understanding Where Peptides Fit in Your Health - Where to Start

Now that you likely know what kind of peptides you want to start with, it's time to understand the best ways to incorporate peptides into your health and wellness regimen.

Depending on your goals, you may be using them to treat acute symptoms like an injury or for long-term wellness like anti-aging.

We'll dive into:

- *The two types of peptide usage (acute and sustained) and examples of each*

- *Deciding where to start*

- *Understanding that everything is connected (lifestyle, nutrition and exercise) and peptides alone are not enough*

- *An intro to combining the different classes of peptides*

- *How to find the right peptide-prescribing physicians, how to engage them, and whether to do it on your own*

We'll use the following tools:

- **Getting Started Infographic** so you can tailor your plan to your regenerative healing goals

- **The Meet Your Goals Peptide Venn Diagram** so you can see how certain classes of peptides overlap and the differences between acute and long-term cycling

- **Your Personal Starting Point** is a tool to document where you're starting and measure your progress.

Module 4: Understanding Peptide Delivery Systems - How to Use the Peptide We've Chosen in the Most Effective Way Possible

Most peptides are administered via some form of injection.

For beginners who are using peptides for the first time, or any veteran biohacker who is experimenting with an unfamiliar peptide, the best approach would be to follow the "**minimum effective dose**" (MED) principle.

In other words, you should start with the lowest dose necessary to produce the desired response/outcome and assess your tolerance to the peptide before you SLOWLY increase the dose.

In other words, start low and go slow...

We'll dive into:

- *The four different ways you can administer peptides and why it matters (hint: buyer beware of nasal sprays in general)*

- *The most effective method(s) of administration*

- *How to safely store, reconstitute, and handle peptides over time*

- *An introduction to dosing (and how to find the best dosage for you as an individual)*

We'll use the following tools:

- **Delivery and Dosage 101** is a video tutorial of how to properly reconstitute and administer peptides

- **Accessing The Peptides** to get you started on **how to purchase them (peptides)** and begin your healing and regenerative journey

- **Doctors that Specialize in Peptides** is a physician vetting checklist so you can find the right doctor for you

Module 5: The Role of Nutrition and Exercise in Your Healing Results

We don't have to tell you that peptides alone won't get you the results you want.

As a health-conscious individual, you know that there's no magic pill when it comes to looking and feeling your best.

In this module, we'll explain the best lifestyle, nutrition, and fitness tips to help you maximize your use of peptides.

We'll dive into:

- *What kind of diet to maintain*

- *The role of insulin-controlled living*

We'll use the following tools:

- **The Critical Role of Nutrition in Your Health:** A guide to maintaining proper nutrition, which is crucial to healing and maintaining optimal health

Module 6: How to Evaluate Results and Adapt Your Protocol

Your response to any therapeutic peptide is 100% individual to you.

You need to do what works FOR YOU, find what works in your favor, and then refine it over time.

As with any health and fitness regimen, you need to monitor, assess, and optimize in order to achieve the results you want.

When you are using therapeutic peptides, you MUST document every single measurable metric so you can have a clear "before-and-after" view of any changes that arise.

In this module, we'll guide you through some of the best practices to help you maintain momentum and ensure that your therapeutic peptide plan is just right for your mind and body's unique needs.

We'll dive into:

- *What N of 1 means*

- *How to accurately evaluate your sensitivity level and monitor how you feel*

- *The super rare side effects to watch for*

- *Setting realistic expectations for yourself*

We'll use the following tools:

- **Benchmarks and Progress Report** so you can benchmark and monitor your progress

- **If this … Then** -- **The Ultimate Guide to Adjusting Your Protocol,** so you can make the right adjustments as necessary

That is all!

We're done with ALL the modules in the courses.

Note that you get all 6 modules just in the **Basic version** of the course.

There's also an **Advanced version** where I have bonus modules that are truly next level.

This is off-the-charts deep intel on how to master the usage of therapeutic peptides.

Nothing else on the planet even comes close.

Now that you have a clear idea about The Peptides Course, if you're ready to buy, then simply visit **pepbk.co/ThePeptidesCourse**.

And don't forget to use the coupon code **PEPTIDESBOOK** at checkout to get your special offer!

ABOUT THE AUTHOR

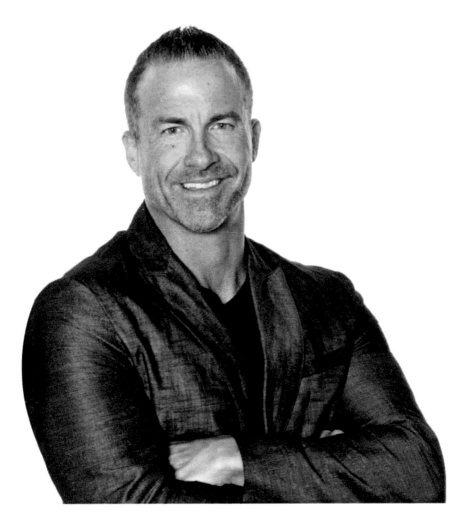

Jay Campbell is a four-time international best-selling author, men's physique champion and founder of the Jay Campbell Brand and Podcast.

Recognized as one of the world's leading experts on hormonal optimization and therapeutic peptides, Jay has dedicated his life to teaching men and women how to #FullyOptimize their health while also instilling the importance of raising their consciousness.

Jay's website[160] (where he's been writing online since 2006) offers some of the most deeply researched articles on the topics of hormone optimization, peptides, fat loss, fitness, and spirituality.

He also hosts the globally acclaimed and Top 50 Medicine Podcast: **The Jay Campbell Podcast** (YouTube[161], Apple[162]).

Jay has been successfully using therapeutic testosterone for more than two decades since the age of 29 and therapeutic peptides since 2004.

One of Jay's primary passions is teaching men and women how to transform their life by using therapeutic testosterone and peptides in the context of long-term health and happiness.

To make his hormonal optimization knowledge scalable, in January of 2022, he launched his online course **TOTDecoded** (TOT stands for Testosterone Optimization Therapy).

---

[160] http://pepbk.co/JayCampbell
[161] http://pepbk.co/YouTube
[162] http://pepbk.co/ApplePodcasts

If you suspect you are suffering from a Testosterone deficiency, you can purchase the course from **pepbk.co/TOTDecoded**.

Use the coupon code **PEPTIDESBOOK** at checkout for a substantial discount off either the Basic or Advanced version.

Jay also has a free email newsletter (read by more than 20,000 subscribers) you can join at **pepbk.co/Newsletter**.

You'll always receive the latest updates and highest-level intel happening in the health optimization world.

The five change-making optimization healthcare books Jay has authored prior to this one are:

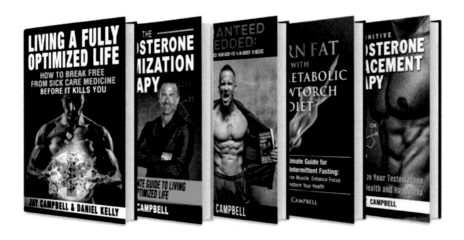

The 2015 released and #1 5-star Rated book of all time on TRT/TOT, **THE Definitive Testosterone Replacement Therapy MANual: How to Optimize Your Testosterone for Lifelong Health and Happiness**[163].

The 2017 Released Intermittent Fasting masterpiece, **The Metabolic Blowtorch Diet-The Ultimate Guide for Optimizing Intermittent Fasting: Burn Fat, Preserve Muscle, Enhance Focus and Transform Your Health**[164].

The #1 overall Men's Health book in 2018, **The Testosterone Optimization Therapy Bible: The Ultimate Guide to Living a Fully Optimized Life**[165].

The 2019 released master treatise on fat loss as an advanced version of the Blowtorch Diet, **Guaranteed Shredded**[166].

The 2019 released book that ties Jay's alchemical mastery altogether, **Living a Fully Optimized Life: How To Break Free from Sick Care Medicine Before It Kills You**[167].

In addition to all of this, Jay has also created his private

---

[163] http://pepbk.co/TheTRTMANual
[164] http://pepbk.co/TheMBTD
[165] http://pepbk.co/TheTOTBible
[166] http://pepbk.co/GuaranteedShredded
[167] http://pepbk.co/LAFOL

online membership group **Fully Optimized Health**[168].

If you're serious about optimizing your hormonal health, losing fat, building strength and muscle, and aging with vigor and vitality (and you want Jay's help with your unique situation), this group is an absolute must.

Join hundreds of CEOs, doctors, fitness competitors, and other highly successful men and women from all walks of life.

Not only will you get to connect directly with them, but you also get direct access to Jay (via his weekly live Ask Me Anything (AMA) calls) and his inner circle of doctors and biohacking experts.

Use the coupon code **PEPTIDESBOOK** at checkout for a Discount on your membership.

At nearly 52 years young (as of Feb 2023), Jay practices what he preaches by maintaining superb physical and mental conditioning year-round.

Creating an anti-fragile and resilient body in the year 2023 is no easy task.

It will not happen by accident or by wishing.

It comes from taking massive action while also

---

[168] http://pepbk.co/FullyOptimizedHealth

harnessing the power of specific medications and supplements shown to slow aging while optimizing physical health.

But since you purchased this book and read all the way to the end...

I have a few more life changing surprises for you...

Those surprises come in the form of 4 amazing bonus chapters

- **How to Heal Like X-Men's Wolverine** (This chapter covers how to maximally supercharge your healing using the therapeutic peptides BPC-157, TB-500, Copper Peptide GHK-Cu while also stacking them with Tesamorelin and Ipamorelin)

- **The God Stack** (All the Golden Age agents I use in 2023 and beyond for molecularly altering my body, mind and spiritual health)

- **What Are Peptide Bioregulators and What Do They Do** (Everything you must know about a new and exciting class of agents that work synergistically with peptides to enhance their effectiveness)

- **Alternate Day Fasting** (Why I use this highly effective nutritional strategy with my private VIP clients to maintain an incredible state of high-performance health)

BONUS CHAPTER
HOW TO HEAL LIKE X-MEN'S WOLVERINE

Without question, the two most well-known peptides to the casual end user are the revolutionary healing peptides BPC-157 and TB-500.

This chapter will cover both of these near-miraculous peptides and the specific role they play in accelerating healing and recovery, along with several others that are often under-appreciated and under-used in the context of bodily repair.

Like all the other peptides covered in this book, there are much deeper scientific dives found on my website for **BPC-157**[169] and **TB-500**[170].

For surgically precise recommendations, here is what you'll receive in this bonus chapter:

- The BEST healing peptides

- How they work in the human body

- The best dose to use them individually

- My fully optimized healing peptide stacks for rapid bodily repair and recovery

---

[169] http://pepbk.co/BPC-157
[170] http://pepbk.co/TB-500

Let's dive right in!

BPC-157

BPC-157[171] is a synthetic 15-amino-acid peptide derived from a peptide called "body protecting compound" (BPC) that is produced in stomach acid (human gastric juice).

Three of its primary mechanisms of action include new blood vessel formation (angiogenesis), the release of the vasodilator nitric oxide[172], and the upregulation of healing factors such as vascular endothelial growth

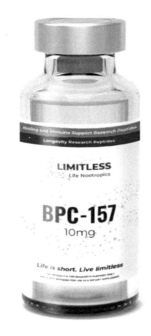

[171] http://pepbk.co/BPC-157
[172] http://pepbk.co/NitricOxide

factor (VEGF).

In several animal studies, and even more anecdotal testimonials from biohackers, the following regenerative effects are consistently observed:

- *Healing of wounds and injuries in muscles, tendons, ligaments, bone, and skin*

- *Increased blood flow to wounded and damaged areas of the body*

- *Protection of your body's organs*

- *Powerful anti-inflammatory responses*

All of the above leads to speeding up the rate of recovery from bodily damage.

Recommended Dosage

 BPC-157 RECOMMENDED DOSAGE

250 mcg injected subcutaneously twice a day.

⚠ IMPORTANT NOTE

I have been using BPC-157 since 2010 for soft tissue sprains and injuries, and the results it is capable of providing are nothing short of miraculous.

Nick Andrews has recently created a new transdermal healing product that will speed the rate of wound healing while also reducing scar tissue formation.

This product will be available thru Limitless Life Nootropics within the very near future.

My wife Monica is having cosmetic surgery to correct capsular contractions from her initial breast augmentation surgery in 2009.

She will be using this new serum, code name 'ReGen' to dramatically speed up her rate of healing.

Stay tuned for more information including before and after of her surgical incisions.

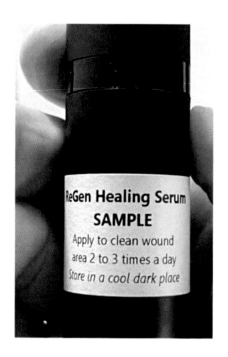

TB-500

TB-500[173] is the active region of a 43-amino-acid peptide called Thymosin Beta-4 (Tβ4) located in every tissue of the human body except for red blood cells.

Tβ4 is secreted by your body's thymus gland as part of its natural healing response, but only so much can be produced (and therefore your rate of recovery from wounds/injuries is limited).

The workaround was to create TB-500, which scientists discovered was the part of the Tβ4 peptide solely

---

[173] http://pepbk.co/TB-500

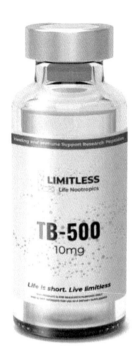

responsible for its healing effects.

These effects are driven by two mechanisms, the first being angiogenesis (very similar to what BPC-157 does, which highlights how critical increased blood flow is for healing any damaged tissue)

Where TB-500 separates itself from BPC-157 is its second mechanism, which involves upregulating a protein called "actin" that promotes the restoration and maintenance of a cell's structure.

This leads to many healing effects that mirror what BPC-157 does:

- *Repairs damage to the heart, skin, tissue, ligaments, and other organs*

- *Boosts immunity*

- *Provides pain relief*

- *Possesses strong anti-inflammatory properties*

Recommended Dosage

 TB-500 RECOMMENDED DOSAGE

2.0-2.5 mg injected subcutaneously or intramuscularly every other day.

 IMPORTANT NOTE

BPC-157 and TB-500 are often stacked together to provide a much faster rate of healing than either used in isolation.

The exact stack and dosages are listed further down in this chapter.

Ipamorelin & Tesamorelin

If you recall the earlier section in this book on fat loss peptides, you already know that **Ipamorelin**[174] is a growth hormone-releasing hormone (GHRH) and **Tesamorelin**[175] is a growth hormone-releasing peptide (GHRP).

They work synergistically to increase the production and release of human growth hormone (hGH).

To use the analogy of a gas tank: Tesamorelin tells your body to fill the tank of hGH all the way to the top, and Ipamorelin tells your body to consume the entire tank of hGH.

Both of these peptides help improve all aspects of tissue regeneration due to hGH's role in the bodily healing process[176].

Recommended Dosage

IPAMORELIN RECOMMENDED DOSAGE

200-300 mcg injected subcutaneously 1-3 times a day.

---

[174] http://pepbk.co/Ipamorelin
[175] http://pepbk.co/Tesamorelin
[176] http://pepbk.co/hGHForRecovery

TESAMORELIN RECOMMENDED DOSAGE

1 mg right before bed yet 90 minutes after your last meal, and 1 mg upon waking yet ideally before exercise (via subcutaneous injection).

GHK-Cu

The copper peptide **GHK-Cu**[177] is useful for far more than reversing hair loss and rejuvenating skin.

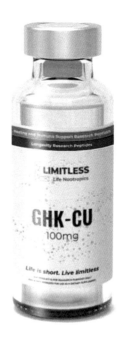

It can stimulate angiogenesis just like BPC-157 and TB-500, but it can also increase collagen production and thereby restore the structural integrity of

---

[177] http://pepbk.co/GHK-Cu

damaged tissues.

Additionally, GHK-Cu can act as a "feedback signal" and instruct the body to simultaneously generate new healthy tissue while removing old damaged tissue.

Other mechanisms of this peptide that take part in speeding up the healing process include:

- *Suppressing chronic inflammation (albeit through separate pathways from TB-500 and BPC-157)*

- *Repairing damaged DNA*

- *Re-igniting the fixing of protective skin barrier proteins*

- *Pain reduction*

GHK-Cu would be best used for soft tissue damage (ex. A sprained/swollen ankle), but would not be useful for something like a broken rib.

Recommended Dosage

 GHK-CU RECOMMENDED DOSAGE

2-4 pumps (0.21 – 0.84 mL) of a 3% topical formulation gently massaged for 30 seconds.

Peptide Healing Stack #1: BPC-157 and TB-500

There are some slight differences between BPC-157 and TB-500 despite their high degree of similarities.

Primarily, BPC-157 is better-suited for treating gastrointestinal issues while TB-500 would be superior for treating heart/muscle and or soft tissue issues.

Outside of this, the two work synergistically to

accelerate the rate of healing even further than either peptide used in isolation.

They both work systemically (i.e. you don't have to inject "locally" into the site of injury itself although there is evidence that injection site healing is more pronounced for specific types of soft tissue injuries).

⚠️ IMPORTANT NOTE

Jay always travels with BPC-157, TB-500 and Thymosin Alpha 1 for protectionary measures in the event of an injury, sickness or bioweapon outbreak.

It is a very prudent course of action when traveling to have access to both peptides for immediate healing and inflammation suppression if/when you or other people sustain a significant injury.

Here's how to use BPC-157 and TB-500 together at the same time[178]:

- *200-750 mcg of BPC-157 injected locally at the site of injury, intramuscularly or subcutaneously, once at morning and once at night.*

- *2.5-3.0 mg of TB-500 injected locally at the site of injury, intramuscularly or subcutaneously, once*

---

[178] http://pepbk.co/TB-500AndBPC-157

a day in the morning or at night (but at the same time as your BPC-157 injection)

- *Continue this protocol for a maximum of 12 weeks or until the injury is 100% healed*

Peptide Healing Stack #2: The Wolverine Protocol

This is the infamous Wolverine Healing Stack featured on my website[179], a massive upgrade to the original "Wolverine Stack" circulating around the Internet.

The "Wolverine Stack" was effectively the first peptide combination I just introduced you to (BPC-157 and TB-500), and nothing more.

My protocol adds on the peptides Tesamorelin, Ipamorelin, and GHK-Cu for extreme speed healing unlike anything seen in the modern medical world.

---

[179] http://pepbk.co/WolverineHealingStack

> ### ⚠️ IMPORTANT NOTE
> One can substitute Genotropin or Norditropin hGH in place of Ipamorelin and Tesamorelin if they are able to locate legally and affordably.

There are just a few caveats you have to know before starting...

Location of injections: Tesamorelin and Ipamorelin are best injected systemically, while the other three peptides (BPC-157, TB-500 and GHK-Cu) are best injected/used locally, ie., at the origin of the injury preferably.

Method of injections: BPC-157 and TB-500 can be injected either intramuscularly or subcutaneously, while Tesamorelin and Ipamorelin are best kept subcutaneous (except GHK-Cu as it can also be administered in the form of a topical cream or serum).

Switching injection sites: Since you're going to be doing a lot of injections per day, make sure you are rotating your injection sites very frequently because it's not practical to perform all of your injections into one part of the body.

Peptide half-lives: The half-lives of these peptides are 30 minutes (Tesamorelin), 2 hours (Ipamorelin), 4 hours (BPC-157), and 1-2 days (TB-500).

This has been factored into how these peptides are spaced out in this protocol.

Without further ado, here are two variations of the Wolverine Protocol you can experiment with:

VARIATION A

- **MORNING**
  - Ipamorelin: 200-300 mcg
  - TB-500: 2.0-2.5 mg
  - BPC-157: 250 mcg
- **EVENING**
  - Tesamorelin: 1 mg
  - BPC-157: 250 mcg
  - GHK-Cu: 2-4 pumps (0.21 – 0.84 mL) of a 3% topical formulation

VARIATION B

- **MORNING**
  - Ipamorelin: 200-300 mcg

- BPC-157: 250 mcg

- GHK-Cu: 2-4 pumps (0.21 – 0.84 mL) of a 3% topical formulation

- **EVENING**

  - Tesamorelin: 1 mg

  - TB-500: 2.0-2.5 mg

  - BPC-157: 250 mcg

Obviously, you will need a heavy amount of self-experimentation and objective self-reflection to determine how to best use my modified Wolverine healing stack.

 IMPORTANT NOTE

Every single peptide in this chapter except for GHK-Cu is officially banned by the World Anti-Doping Association (WADA) under one of the following two categories:

- S0 - Unapproved substances
- S2 - Peptide hormones, growth factors, related substances and mimetics

Please keep this in mind if you are a competitive athlete of any kind.

BONUS CHAPTER
THE "GOD STACK" FOR
FULLY OPTIMIZED HEALTH

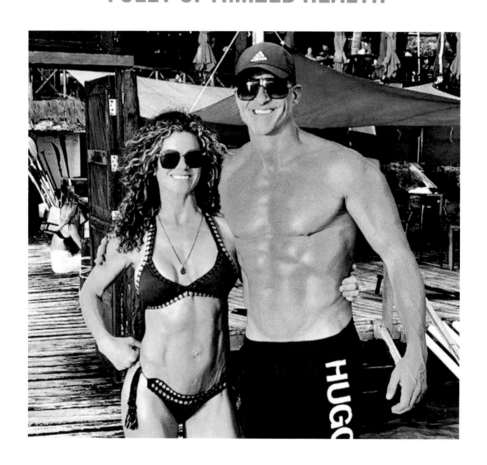

"God Stack" Agent #1:
Therapeutic Testosterone

If you're a long-time reader of my content, I don't have

to explain why testosterone holds the #1 spot[180].

As I've explained everywhere (in my blog, podcasts, and books), the rapid decline of the average male's natural testosterone levels still rages on.

We can certainly continue to blame endocrine-disrupting chemicals, but by and large, the pandemic-induced "work at home" lifestyles have exponentially increased the incidence of unhealthy habits.

Higher sugar and alcohol consumption, chronic stress levels rising, increased body fat gain, decreased physical movement... I could go on forever.

Testosterone has been — and will always be — the lifeblood molecule and foundation for every single facet of male and female health:

- *Stronger natural immunity against disease*

- *Increased libido*

- *Elevated social status*

- *Protection against mood disorders like depression*

- *More lean muscle gain*

Long story short: Testosterone optimization therapy is a game-changing, lifesaving therapy for men and women

---

[180] http://pepbk.co/Testosterone

who have a clinical need for it via symptoms first and blood work second.

It is imperative (if possible, depending on what country you reside) one works with an experienced doctor who knows how to optimize and balance hormonal levels.

Recommended Dosage

Everybody's weekly dosage will be customized to their health situation as we are all N-of-1 and biochemically unique.

It is highly recommended one chooses one of the two methods listed below as their preferred therapeutic testosterone delivery system to ensure optimal results:

THERAPEUTIC TESTOSTERONE RECOMMENDED DOSAGE

- **Subcutaneous daily or EOD (every other day) injection of a testosterone ester such as cypionate or propionate:** I spent 18 years using every-other-day injections for a total of 150 mg of injectable testosterone per week. Normal weekly dosages should not exceed 200 mg except in rare occurrences.

- **A compounded trans-scrotal testosterone cream:** 200 mg of testosterone per gram of cream 200 mg/g with Versa base (or HRT base) applied 1-2x/day to a clean, shaven, and dry scrotum

DO NOT use a "gel" on your scrotum because it will burn your skin.

If it's not a compounded cream, and it's not at the 200 mg/g concentration, you won't properly optimize your testosterone levels and are unlikely to maximize the effects desired.

Hopefully one day we'll have an oral version (YES, A TRULY EFFICACIOUS ORAL PHARMA TEST PRODUCT).

A "real-life testosterone booster" unlike all the fake bullshit products men continue to be ripped off by.

A product that provides all the benefits of injections and/or transdermal delivery systems equally as well, if not better.

For a comprehensive explanation of therapeutic testosterone, read my best-selling book **Testosterone Optimization Therapy Bible**[181].

Or my constantly updated, comprehensive online course on the topic: **TOT Decoded**[182].

---

[181] http://pepbk.co/TheTOTBible
[182] http://pepbk.co/TOTDecoded

"God Stack" Agent #2: Desiccated Thyroid

Desiccated thyroid[183] is my go-to for keeping my thyroid gland in an optimized state.

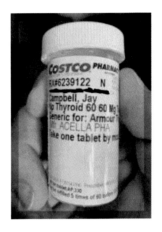

The human thyroid gland is a small yet powerful bodily organ responsible for regulating metabolic rate.

It is also responsible for other important bodily processes such as heat production and heart rate.

Reduced production of thyroid hormones (T1, T2, T3, T4) as one ages often leads to unwanted side effects such as hair thinning, loss of cognition, and a seeming inability to lose body fat.

But where many people go wrong is using extreme low calorie crash diets.

These diets crash thyroid hormone production (most female fitness competitors do this regularly) relative to one's ideal body weight.

---

[183] http://pepbk.co/DesiccatedThyroid

Many men and women also abuse the use of synthetic thyroid hormone medications (Cytomel or Synthroid, which only target T3 and T4 thyroid hormones) to artificially increase their body's fat-burning rate while in a caloric deficit (much in the same way bodybuilders abuse anabolic steroids via supraphysiological doses).

Oftentimes this causes long term, if not permanent, thyroid dysfunction.

This is where desiccated thyroid comes into the picture:

It's a naturally derived mixture of all four major thyroid hormones (T1, T2, T3 and T4) that DOES NOT interfere with your body's regular thyroid hormone production.

The side effects are far fewer compared to using synthetic T3 or T4.

They are just as useful for people suffering from inferior thyroid hormone regulation.

Recommended Dosage

DESICCATED THYROID RECOMMENDED DOSAGE

30-60 mg (I prefer Armour Thyroid) taken 1-2/xday, once in the morning while fasted and a second dose in the mid-afternoon if desired.

Please make sure (a) you have a CLINICAL need for desiccated thyroid, and (b) you are regularly doing the blood work measuring the biomarkers described within the reference article.

"God Stack" Agent #3: Metformin

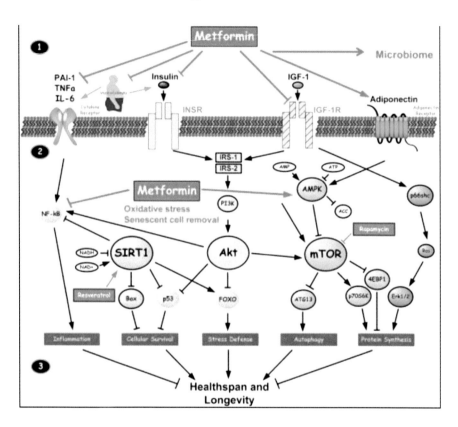

Discovered in 1922, we've had this plant-derived medication available to us for exactly 100 years.

It is primarily used in adults suffering from Type II Diabetes as a medication for increasing insulin sensitivity, lowering systemic inflammation, and decreasing glucose absorption.

Metformin[184] does much more for humans living an

---

[184] http://pepbk.co/Metformin

insulin-controlled life who also desire fully optimized health.

It is proven to extend lifespan and provides multiple mechanisms for the following biological effects:

- *Anti-cancer activity*

- *Protection against cognitive decline*

- *Improvement of gut health by increasing akkermansia formation*

- *Improvement of cardiovascular protection*

There's no question that Metformin is a "therapeutic wonder drug" for enhancing human longevity and performance.

But sadly, the past 60 years have shown Metformin is still surrounded by constant misinformation.

This is despite being safer and far more extensively studied than 99% of all other pharmaceutical drugs.

Much of the false intel can be explained by the following:

- *Misinformation about it causing renal issues in healthy people still propagated in medical schools*

- *Inappropriate dosages used*

- *Misleading context about the human populations used (almost always these studies are done in diseased and co-morbid patient population groups) to make certain conclusions in select studies*

- *A failure to read the fine print of what regulatory agencies have said about it*

- *A complete misunderstanding of basic pharmacokinetics and pharmacodynamics*

There are only two conditions where Metformin's benefits do not outweigh the risks:

- *Your kidneys are SEVERELY impaired (if only slightly, there are many instances where Metformin is still clinically OK and optimal assuming patient lifestyle modulation)*

- *You are a top 1% powerlifter/strength athlete competing in the most elite events the world has to offer, due to slight reduction of maximal power output from M-tor regulation*

If you must ASK yourself whether you are an elite-level athlete or not, there's a near-100% chance you belong to the latter.

Recommended Dosage

 METFORMIN RECOMMENDED DOSAGE

500-1000 mg 2x/day for men, 250-500 mg 2x/day for women.

Take the first dose in the early morning while fasted, and the second dose right before dinner.

As always, start low and go slow when titrating your dosage up or down.

"God Stack" Agent #4: Melanotan 1

This peptide[185] is singlehandedly the best pharma compound in existence for consciousness expansion and melanin boosting (to enhance tanning).

Ancestral researchers and shamans always knew about the connection between melanin and vibrating at a higher frequency.

The extremely important work of Dr. Frank Barr regarding melanin receptor complexes and their overall

---

[185] http://pepbk.co/Melanotan1

organizing ability in living systems[186] was also instrumental in validating this connection.

Melanotan 1 has helped me attain a much more still state of mind where I am calmer and more grounded, certainly more than anything I have achieved through intense meditation alone.

There are indeed other health benefits to be conferred, such as:

- *Getting an even yet not-too-dark skin tan (via increased melanin production)*

- *Treating skin diseases such as vitiligo*

- *Protecting against neuroinflammation and UV-induced damage to your DNA*

- *Optimizing spiritual health better than any other pharmaceutical agent*

The only major downside is that Melanotan 1 is only available as a prescription drug (under the name "afamelanotide") for treating erythropoietic protoporphyria.

As such, it is no longer procured cheaply from research chemical companies as it was 10-15 years ago (15 vials at $10/vial would last most users a YEAR).

---

[186] http://pepbk.co/Melanin

You now need a doctor's script and the financial means to pay a significant amount for a month's supply.

Recommended Dosage

MELATONAN 1 RECOMMENDED DOSAGE

0.25 mg injected subcutaneously 1-2x/week for a maximum of 8 months consistently before cycling off for 3-4 months (if you use it for skin tanning, you'll need a slightly higher dose alongside regular sunlight exposure)

What About Melanotan 2?

While I've previously written about the peptide Melanotan 2[187] and its health benefits, I no longer recommend it as I believe it has zero purpose.

If you read the full article, I discuss Melanotan 2's nasty habit of making your skin Oompa-Loompa orange.

Not a healthy browner tan skin tone.

You literally look like an unsightly cartoon character.

---

[187] http://pepbk.co/Melanotan2

While both Melanotan 1 and Melanotan 2 produce a "browning" of melanin, Melanotan 2 has a disturbing effect of taking the act of skin tanning a few steps too far.

(There's a reason it's called "The Barbie Drug" - look up what happens to people who abuse it).

Whereas Melanotan 1 will give you the desired 1-2 shades of darker color you're looking for (relative to the natural levels of melanin you possess).

But there are three other side effects of Melanotan 2 which I believe are far more severe and more frequent than what's being reported...

- *Mole formation and darkening, which may accelerate the development of life-threatening skin cancer depending on your genetics*

- *Increased erectile function to the point of priapism (i.e., an erection lasting several hours to the point of extreme discomfort and pain)*

- *Feeling nauseous*

The last one is especially pertinent to me as I was foolish enough to combine Melanotan 1 and a micro dose of Melanotan 2 prior to a trip I recently took to Miami as I was prepping for a photo shoot to promote the **Positive Muscular Failure course**[188].

What happens is that you feel fine after your morning injection, but five hours later you feel like throwing up.

This effect kicked in while I was mid-flight and I spent most of the flight in the airplane bathroom bent over the toilet (i.e., dry heaving, where you feel like puking, but nothing comes out).

Not anything anyone wants to experience if possible.

In summation: My article on Melanotan 2[189] still stands with respect to scientific accuracy and completeness, but in practice I am no longer recommending it.

"God Stack" Agent #5: Microdose of Human Growth Hormone (Genotropin)

Human growth hormone (hGH)[190], not to sound like a cliche, literally does damn near everything.

From the time you are born and throughout adulthood, it helps grow your muscles and bones, regulates the metabolism of fats and carbohydrates, and helps to maintain healthy body composition.

---

[188] http://pepbk.co/PMFTraining
[189] http://pepbk.co/Melanotan2
[190] http://pepbk.co/hGH

It also happens to be a frequently used weapon in the lives of people focused on life extension and age regression.

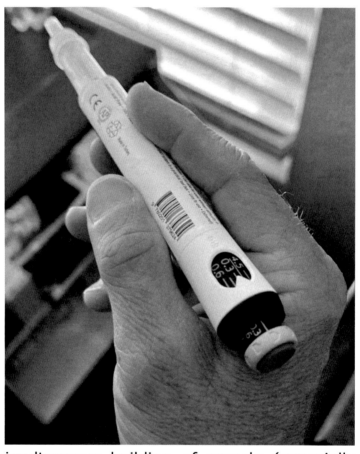

The simultaneous building of muscle (especially when combined with therapeutic testosterone) and shedding of stubborn body fat makes it an ideal choice for muscle gain without the normal body fat acclimation.

As I mention in the reference article, there are numerous agents and peptides which increase the production, secretion, and "pulse" of hGH.

But if you're going to use hGH, my favorite is Pfizer's Genotropin[191] prescribed to children and adults with growth hormone deficiency:

> "Genotropin is a recombinant human growth hormone (also called somatropin).
>
> It has the same structure as natural human growth hormone which is needed for bones and muscles to grow.
>
> It also helps your fat and muscle tissues to develop in the right amounts.
>
> Recombinant means it is made using bacteria instead of being taken out of human or animal tissue."

True pharma-grade hGH is what I call "the nectar of the gods" for anti-aging.

Not all "Pharma-Grade" hGH is created equally, however, and experienced users of "other brands" will be able to understand this distinction once they've used Genotropin.

Norditropin hGH from Nordisk is also a high quality hGH that compares similarly to Genotropin from Pfizer.

---

[191] http://pepbk.co/Genotropin

When hGH is micro-dosed appropriately, it is a life-extension agent that DOES NOT interfere with your body's natural production of hGH while sleeping.

(There are people who will debate this statement but it's up to the end user to determine the truth via IGF-1 laboratory readings upon use and discontinuing of use).

Recommended Dosage

 GENOTROPIN RECOMMENDED DOSAGE

0.75-2.0 IUs a day injected subcutaneously and best taken in the early morning while fasted (avoiding food 30 minutes before injecting and 1.5 hours post injection).

I recommend women start with the minimal dose possible on the pen (0.75 IUs) and titrate upward based on subcutaneous water retention.

I normally take 1.5 IUs from Monday-Friday and cycle off during the weekends (Most women can get by with dosing 0.75-1 IUs in the same way).

I also perform fasted cardio within 15-30 minutes of dosing for maximal fat loss.

"God Stack" Agent #6: Tesofensine

Once a failed pharmaceutical candidate for treating Alzheimer's and Parkinson's, the unintended "side effect" of rapid weight loss turned Tesofensine[192] into a superstar candidate for getting shredded to the bone.

But what makes it unique from other fat loss agents is its multi-pronged approach:

- *Reduced physical hunger AND reduced mental cravings via reuptake of dopamine and serotonin*

- *Increased basal metabolic rate (BMR) likely through noradrenaline reuptake*

- *Lowered levels of risk-associated biomarkers such as "bad" cholesterol*

- *Sustained weight loss (i.e., fat tissue loss, waist reduction) that proves superior to existing weight loss drugs on the market*

It also happens to increase BDNF production[193], strengthening your connection to divinity (source consciousness) while elevating your mood and

---

[192] http://pepbk.co/Tesofensine
[193] http://pepbk.co/BDNF

increasing overall cognition.

Improved production of BDNF also provides better long-term memory, a clearer mind, a stronger ability to focus on difficult tasks, and increases the speed and rate of learning.

While most fat loss agents only focus on 1-2 of the four aspects related to fat loss I just discussed, Tesofensine does them all and does each one exceptionally.

I've been using this drug since late February 2022, and I am the leanest I have ever been with the least amount of work.

If you've ever seen the pictures I took for the **Positive Muscular Failure course**[194], that's the power of Tesofensine in action.

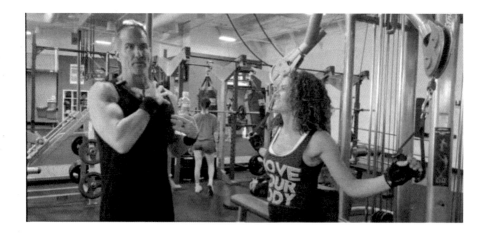

---

[194] http://pepbk.co/PMFTraining

Tesofensine is available to purchase via **Limitless Life Nootropics**[195].

Don't forget to use code *JAY15* for 15% off your order!

Your other option is to procure compounded Tesofensine via a script from a doctor[196].

Depending on the doctor or clinic prescribing you Tesofensine, you may be looking at significantly higher cost than purchasing directly from a research chemical company like Limitless.

Recommended Dosage

TESOFENSINE RECOMMENDED DOSAGE

One 0.5 mg tablet first thing in the morning fasted every day.

The research shows this medication continues to produce results 6 months into use, so my recommendation is to use it during the months of the year you want to remain the leanest.

[195] http://pepbk.co/LimitlessLifeNootropics
[196] http://pepbk.co/MedicalHealthInstitute

After using it for close to one year and withdrawing "cold turkey" for 2 months, I have not experienced any symptoms or side effects.

IMO, this proves it is well tolerated and one does not develop any dependance over a longer course of administration.

"God Stack" Agent #7: Tirzepatide

Tirzepatide[197] is what many consider to be the successor to Semaglutide[198] when it comes to superior weight loss and appetite suppression.

(This peptide was developed by Eli Lilly and is marketed under the brand name "Mounjaro")

Tirzepatide is a synthetic modification of a hormone peptide known as glucose-dependent insulinotropic peptide (GIP), which carries out the following functions when attached to its receptor:

- *Induce insulin secretion*

- *Increases insulin sensitivity*

- *Improves lipid metabolism and triglyceride*

---

[197] http://pepbk.co/Tirzepatide
[198] http://pepbk.co/SemaglutideAndAOD-9604

clearance

- *Lowers bodyweight*

Not only does Tirzepatide target GIP's receptors, but it also targets the same receptors of glucagon-like peptide-1 (GLP-1) as Semaglutide does.

GLP-1's biological functions[199] are highly similar yet somewhat different from those of GIP:

- *Suppresses glucagon secretion*

- *Blunts appetite (giving you the feeling of being full)*

- *Stimulates insulin release from pancreas to lower blood glucose levels*

- *Delays gastric emptying*

So, while Semaglutide only targeted GLP-1 receptors, Tirzepatide goes after the receptors of both GLP-1 AND GIP.

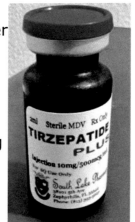

And across numerous Phase 3 trials[200], Tirzepatide was superior to placebo and any other equivalent drug such as Semaglutide when faced head-to-head in both diabetic and

---

[199] http://pepbk.co/GLP-1
[200] http://pepbk.co/TirzepatidePhase3Trials

non-diabetic obese patients.

Specifically, patients found themselves feeling much fuller and losing more body weight within the same period.

Researchers also observed big reductions in glycosylated hemoglobin (HbA1c), and an equivalent (if not lower) severity and frequency of side effects in comparison to Semaglutide and other GLP-1 receptor agonists.

Unfortunately, due to Tirzepatide's status as a prescription drug, it is difficult to find online.

Many compounding pharmacies (and research chemical companies) are now looking at adding additional agents to Tirzepatide in order to not violate the patent of the original formulation "Mounjaro".

IMPORTANT NOTE

I've recently come to find out there is a third-generation drug in the pipeline that may be significantly better than Tirzepatide.

A medication which may have already ascended Tirzepatide with respect to faster body fat loss, greater metabolic uncoupling and stronger appetite reduction.

Eli Lilly is currently developing a drug named "Retatrutide" (code name "LY3437943") which is in Phase II clinical trials.

What makes Retatrutide unique is that it targets THREE receptors.

Semaglutide targeted the receptor glucagon-like peptide-1 (GLP-1), and Tirzepatide targeted both the GLP-1 receptor and glucose-dependent insulinotropic peptide (GIP) receptor.

This potentially all-powerful weight loss drug tackles GLP-1 and GIP receptors while also targeting the body's glucagon receptors.

Supposedly, this three-pronged approach gives the drug a **DIRECT effect on energy expenditure**[201] (unlike its predecessors).

We effectively have a lowering of appetite from GLP-1, improved fat clearance with GIP, and a higher metabolic rate (uncoupling) with the glucagon receptor.

Look at this early preclinical study[202] done in mice and tell me your mind isn't BLOWN AWAY:

---

[201] http://pepbk.co/RetatrutideStudy
[202] http://pepbk.co/RetatrutidePreclinicalStudy

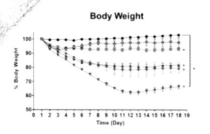

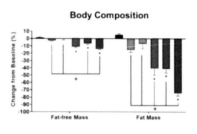

- LY3437943 shows superior weight loss compared to selective GLP-1 RA and dual agonists (e.g. Cotadutide or LY3305677 [dual GLP-1R/GCGR agonist] or tirzepatide [dual GIPR/GLP-1R agonist])
- The weight loss observed is mainly driven by fat mass loss (~80%)

Tirzepatide is in blue and Retatrutide is in red — not only is the total weight loss significantly larger, but most of the weight loss is PURE BODY FAT.

In a Phase 1 clinical trial[203], Retatrutide led to a mean body weight loss of up to 8.96 kg after a study period of 12 weeks.

To put this in context: When Tirzepatide was evaluated in a Phase 3 clinical trial[204], the body weight loss ranged from 7.0 kg to 9.5 kg after a study period of 40 weeks.

Although this early data is incredible, and on top of needing Phase 2 and Phase 3 trials before official FDA approval, we still need to see Retatrutide go head-to-head against Semaglutide and Tirzepatide in order to compare the weight loss and changes in obesity-related biomarkers directly.

---

[203] http://pepbk.co/RetatrutidePhase1Trial
[204] http://pepbk.co/RetatrutidePhase3Trial

I'll also need to find a way to access this peptide so I can try it out for myself (As always, IT IS in the works and stay tuned).

The future of weight loss medications has never looked brighter, especially given the many failed drugs[205] that came before it.

Recommended Dosage

 TIRZEPATIDE RECOMMENDED DOSAGE

For a reasonably **healthy person** (not obese), 2.5 mg injected subcutaneously once a week for a month (4 weeks total), and then increased to 5 mg once per week for the second month (Although for already lean individuals, 2.5 mg is a highly effective dosage that can be continued without increase).

For **obese people** in serious need of glycemic control due to diabetes, keep increasing the dose in 2.5 mg increments every four weeks but never exceed 15 mg injected subcutaneously once a week.

---

[205] http://pepbk.co/FailedWeightLossDrugs

Understanding the potential of all these current and future amazing fat loss peptide medications to choose, I recommended working with an experienced doctor/clinic who will not only write a script for you but be your personal guide on the path to becoming fully optimized.

As of December 2022, and going forward, my preferred health optimization clinic is **Medical Health Institute**[206] and their owners Carlos and Michael Bertonatti.

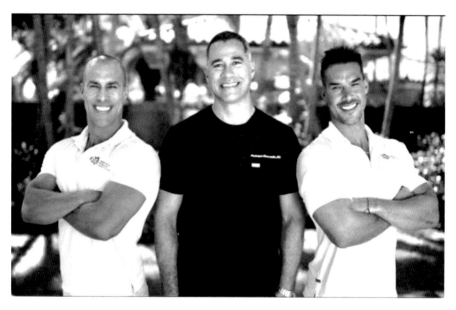

Their awesome medical staff, including physicians Dr. Rudolph Eberwein M.D.[207] and Dr. Amy Wecker, are both highly skilled in helping their patients become hormonally optimized.

[206] http://pepbk.co/MedicalHealthInstitute
[207] reberwein@yahoo.com

They are also experts with prescribing therapeutic peptides and will reliably script the agents written about in this book (when there is an indicated clinical need) for the same purposes.

"God Stack" Agent #8: Melatonin

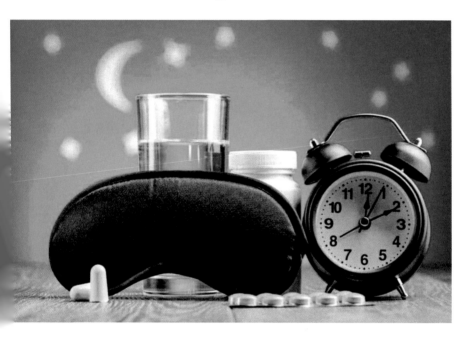

Melatonin's anti-inflammatory and antioxidative properties, combined with its over-the-counter availability, have always made it a highly recommended and useful agent alongside ascorbic acid (Vitamin C).

But emerging research[208] suggests it is far more useful for many other applications:

---

[208] http://pepbk.co/MelatoninResearch

"Some studies have shown that melatonin may also be effective in breast cancer, fibrocystic breast diseases, and colon cancer.

Melatonin has been shown to modify immunity, the stress response, and certain aspects of the aging process; some studies have demonstrated improvements in sleep disturbances and "sundowning" in patients with Alzheimer's disease.

The antioxidant role of melatonin may be of potential use for conditions in which oxidative stress is involved in the pathophysiologic processes.

The multiplicity of actions and variety of biological effects of melatonin suggest the potential for a range of clinical and wellness-enhancing uses."

You clearly won't go wrong using Melatonin to reduce jet lag symptoms and improve all aspects of deep sleep (falling asleep faster, staying asleep, resetting your circadian rhythm, etc.).

There is not much more to say here, other than I've grown very fond of this agent for the reasons stated above.

Recommended Dosage

 MELATONIN RECOMMENDED DOSAGE

10-30 mg taken 90 minutes before bed (according to recent research, higher doses of Melatonin appear safe for human consumption).

Experiment first by starting low and going slow regarding adjusting your dosage upward.

BONUS CHAPTER
WHAT ARE PEPTIDE BIOREGULATORS AND WHAT DO THEY DO?

After writing so extensively about virtually every peptide in existence[209], I've discovered a brand-new class of therapeutic peptides that are mostly obscured from the west.

One hidden away from the Western hemisphere but very much popular in the motherland of Russia.

They're known as peptide bioregulators and to this day you won't hear about them unless you're "in the know".

As you'll soon find out, they are very different from mainstream-type medications, hormones, anesthetics, and even common injectable peptides such as BPC-157[210] and TB-500[211].

And due to their unique mechanism of action, these "bioregulators" can even be combined with traditional peptides for an unbelievably synergistic effect.

Keep reading and you'll see why I'm excited about what the future has in store for peptide bioregulators!

---

[209] http://pepbk.co/Peptides
[210] http://pepbk.co/BPC-157
[211] http://pepbk.co/TB-500

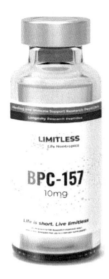
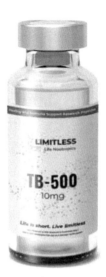

In order to explain what peptide bioregulators are, we need to set in stone some very hard definitions.

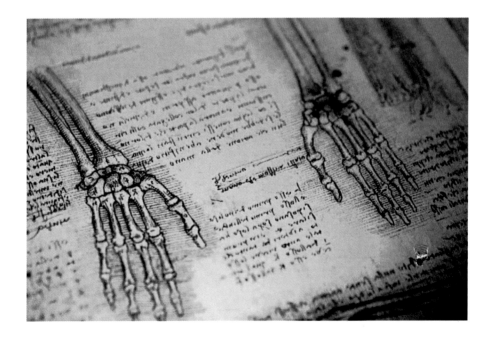

There are too many articles on the Internet that do not very clearly differentiate between peptides and peptide bioregulators.

While peptide bioregulators are technically peptides, they are very distinct from traditional peptides and therefore the two terms cannot be used interchangeably.

Let's go over the differences that demonstrate why bioregulators are their own unique class of peptides...

Peptides vs. Peptide Bioregulators: Method of Administration

When you hear me or anybody in the Western hemisphere use the word "peptide", we are referring to an injectable bioactive peptide (or sublingual/intranasal for select peptides).

Keep in mind this does not necessarily mean a given peptide is a bioregulator, especially when you are using technical language[212]:

- Peptide: A molecule formed by the linking together of two or more amino acids (up to 50)

---

[212] http://pepbk.co/ListOfBioregulatorPeptides

- <u>Polypeptide</u>: A string of more than 50 amino acids linked together

- <u>Protein</u>: Two or more polypeptide chains linked together for a specific function

- <u>Bioregulator</u>: Chemical compounds produced by cells in one part of an organism that have profound regulatory effects on biological processes within the organism

In the Eastern hemisphere, specifically the Middle East and Russia, when they use the word "peptide" they are including both bioregulators and traditional peptides such as BPC- 157.

HOWEVER, in the context of peptide bioregulators specifically, they are distinct from normal peptides in they are orally active and taken in the form of a capsule/tablet.

This is crucial because any "peptide" commonly known in Western culture has zero functional oral activity and will get destroyed by the stomach[213]:

> *"Since proteins are an important part of the diet, the stomach and intestines harbor countless enzymes that break peptide bonds. No medication based on unmodified peptides would have a*

---

[213] http://pepbk.co/OralPeptides

chance to survive the passage through the gastrointestinal tract.

Yet even when appropriately modified peptide compounds make it through the stomach intact, another hurdle awaits them: The cells of the intestinal walls prevent their absorption into the blood.

That is why these kinds of active agents are generally only administered by injection."

There are two reasons why peptide bioregulators are only available in oral formulation within Russia:

1. Keeping peptide bioregulators as capsules/tablets allowed manufacturers to label them as "supplements" and avoid unnecessary regulatory hurdles

2. For whatever mechanistic reason related to molecular similarity and your body "knowing" what to do with them, peptide bioregulators just happen to be orally active.

Although bioregulators may get metabolized in the stomach (not completely), enough of the active ingredient gets shuttled to the relevant biological system.

Peptides vs. Peptide Bioregulators: Selectivity

While traditional peptides tend to almost always be systemic (i.e., affecting the entire body), peptide bioregulators are systems specific.

In other words, bioregulators are naturally selective and will get shuttled to their associated organ instead of going everywhere in the body (more on that later).

Almost nobody understands the difference unless they use and study both classes of peptides.

Therefore, I'm going out of my way to make these differences very clear to everyone who reads this bonus chapter.

Peptides vs. Peptide Bioregulators: Speed of Action

Traditional peptides such as GHK-Cu will have a rapid observable effect and it won't take long for you to notice changes.

Peptide bioregulators are the opposite: Excluding exceptions, you will see results over no sooner than 4 weeks and there are no rapid observable effects.

Due to requiring sustained use for an extended period to see significant benefits, you must "start low and go slow" with your dosage while exercising patience.

Peptides vs. Peptide Bioregulators: History & Availability

Unlike traditional peptides that have an entire century of history and discovery stories ranging from all around the world, the history of peptide bioregulators is exclusively limited to the boundaries of Russia[214]:

> "...the first peptide bioregulators were developed back in the 70's of the last century in the Military Medical Academy named after Kirov, and then at the St. Petersburg Institute of Bioregulation and Gerontology the scientists continued their study and the creation of new peptide drugs.
>
> All peptide bioregulators are patented in the Russian Federation and in the leading countries of Europe and the USA (more than 200 patents)."

---

[214] http://pepbk.co/TrofimovaInterview

The bioregulators are largely the brainchild of Dr. Vladmir Khavinson, who you may remember was responsible for spearheading the research into the life-extension properties of Epitalon[215] and Thymalin[216].

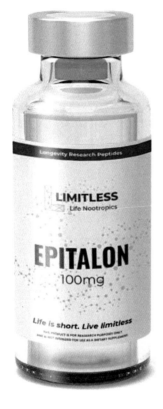 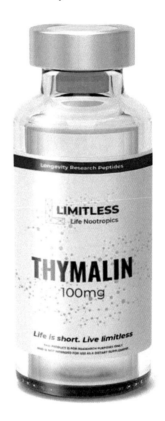

For that reason, you may seem some people refer to this specific group of peptides as "Khavinson bioregulators".

It also explains why peptide bioregulators are relatively unheard of in the West.

---

[215] http://pepbk.co/Epitalon
[216] http://pepbk.co/Thymalin

The Russians have patent protection on all their development work and their research is very closed off to the outside world (unless you can fluently read and speak Russian).

Not to mention the makeup of peptide bioregulators, as you'll see later, means they cannot be easily commercialized by Big Pharma companies.

How Do Peptide Bioregulators Work?

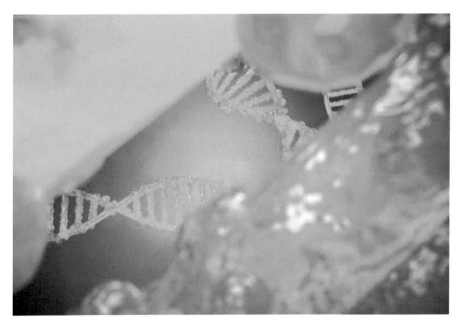

Now that we understand what peptide bioregulators are and what they are not, let's dig deeper and describe how they work.

As the name implies, bioregulators are natural substances in our body that attempt to return our systems back to a healthy state of biological equilibrium.

They participate in tissue repair by interacting with our cellular DNA directly and accelerating the process of protein synthesis[217]:

> "...cells produce low-molecular-weight compounds of a peptide nature, which provide the intercellular transfer of certain information encoded in the amino acid sequence and conformational modifications, thus regulating proliferation, differentiation, and intercellular interactions"

> "... bioregulators participate in the regulation of gene expression and protein synthesis. This fact is in accordance with the concept of the regulation of cascade peptide of physiological functions of the organism"

> "Short peptides are able to interact with DNA regions and thus affect the genome condition and consequently the synthesis of certain proteins, including those that control the physiological functions of the organism"

---

[217] http://pepbk.co/PeptideBioregulatorsStudy

While a healthy biological system will work to increase endogenous levels of peptide bioregulators over time, they are much like naturally produced traditional peptides in that their production decreases with age and/or inflammation and disease.

Which is why the logical approach is to re-introduce these peptide bioregulators through an outside source.

But if you recall what I said earlier, the selective nature of peptide bioregulators means they will ONLY restore biological function/activity from the same organ they were originally extracted from.

In other words, you can't use bioregulators from your cartilage to restore cells in your retina!

So, you need to be intentional and purposeful when you are ingesting them.

And although this won't matter much in the grand scheme of things, some scientists and vendors insist there are three specific types of peptide bioregulators[218]:

1. Cytamins: bioregulators purified from cattle organs that are a complex mixture of nucleoproteins, amino acids, and vitamins

2. Cytomaxes: bioregulators isolated from animal

---

[218] http://pepbk.co/TypesOfPeptideBioregulators

organs/tissues that contain low-molecular-weight peptide fractions (i.e., a pure peptide instead of a mixture of components)

3. Cytogens: bioregulators that are synthetically made in a lab from amino acids, usually forming a peptide that's 3 amino acids long, based on select regions of polypeptides extracted from animal organs/tissues that have biological activity one is looking for

Let's see some examples of bioregulators in action!

Uses of Peptide Bioregulators

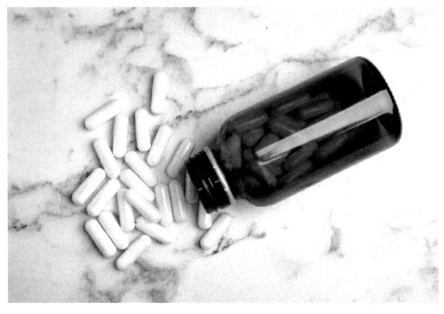

As much as I like to harp on America's "sick care

system"[219], we have the money and the manpower to run our own research and fully test these peptide bioregulators for ourselves.

All supposed effects are speculative due to most positive data coming from the anecdotal testimonials of biohackers and ordinary people.

Additionally, there are way too many peptide bioregulators for me to cover due to their selective nature.

Just look at how many of them this Russian vendor[220] is selling — I'd end up writing a book if I wrote about each one of them.

Testes, thyroid, muscles, heart, bladder, retina, pancreas... if there's an organ system in your body, there is one or more bioregulators for it.

So, with those two things in mind, I'm going to cover three peptide bioregulators I found interesting.

All the information below is taken directly from a book called **The Peptide Bioregulator Revolution**[221], a very dense 58-page book that will tell you way more about bioregulators than I ever could.

---

[219] http://pepbk.co/ThePriceWePay
[220] http://pepbk.co/Rupharma
[221] http://pepbk.co/ThePeptideBioregulatorRevolution

Just consider this as a fraction of what is possible with these Golden Age compounds!

CERLUTEN

- Extract from young animals' brain tissue

- Boosts several brain functions that play a role in preventing brain failure due to trauma

- May reduce side effects of medications affecting the brain

- Recommended to take two capsules daily for a month, and do another cycle 3-6 months later

GOTRATIX

- Mixture of peptides extracted from young animals' tricep muscle

- Regulates muscle metabolism, improves adaptation to exercise

- Useful for muscle weakness and for athletes seeking boosts in physical performance

- May lower muscle fatigue and shorten recovery time

VESUGEN

- Synthetically created tripeptide (lysine, glutamine, asparagine)

- Used to treat heart and vascular conditions

- May indirectly improve skin metabolism via regulation of blood circulation in capillaries

- Could help reduce levels of very low-density lipoproteins (VLDL)

Unfortunately, **I do not know of a 100% reliable source to buy high-quality peptide bioregulators.**

Due to my lack of experience using them, I won't recommend any vendor over another.

Dr Bill Lawrence is clearly the USA's leading researcher on bioregulators.

He is a longevity researcher amid a 3-year trial using bioregulator peptides to see how they influence biological age vs chronological age.

This is understood by measuring telomeres and measuring DNA methylation using the Horvath DNA methylation clock[222].

I highly recommend viewing this two-part podcast

---

[222] http://pepbk.co/DNAMethylation

Natalie Niddam did with Dr Bill Lawrence (Part 1[223] and Part 2[224]) to gain a much greater understanding about peptide bioregulators.

If you choose to use peptide bioregulators, make sure you use them specifically to address the root cause of your problem(s).

If you are interested in using a Peptide and Bioregulator stack designed specifically to help heal and recover from 'experimental gene therapy' you might have been exposed to, please visit my website and **read this article**[225].

⚠ IMPORTANT NOTE

There are companies in the marketplace that now provide analysis of human biological age.

One of them is **TruDiagnostic** whose founder, Ryan Smith, is a good friend of mine.

TruDiagnostic provides the most advanced epigenetic analysis for research and discovery.

The novel DNA biomarker uses markers on your DNA called methylation to predict your age.

---

[223] http://pepbk.co/BioregulatorLongevity1
[224] http://pepbk.co/BioregulatorLongevity2
[225] http://pepbk.co/GeneTherapy

Your biological age is more accurate at predicting health span (how healthy you are) and lifespan (how long you will live) than any previous molecular biomarker.

Epigenetic Methylation is a promising biomarker of the future, but in order to read the information found in our unique methylation, we must be able to interpret it.

TruDiagnostic's CLIA certified laboratory specializes in DNA methylation and generating new algorithms to interpret this data for health insights.

If you are interested in measuring your own unique biological age, **click here**[226] and use code JC50 to take $50 OFF.

---

[226] http://pepbk.co/TruDiagnostic

BONUS CHAPTER
FASTING EVERY OTHER DAY (ALTERNATE DAY FASTING)

If you can fast for 20 hours a day, three to four times a week, you will radically alter your body composition.

Combining these types of long fast intervals with the agents I've mentioned in this book GUARANTEES supremely low levels of body fat in both men and women.

Men can indeed get down to the single digits (5-7% body fat) while women who get shredded should never go below 12-14% (due to internal fat storage for bio evolutionary reasons i.e., giving birth).

As I wrote in my book **The Metabolic Blowtorch Diet**[227], there are numerous proven health benefits of fasting:

- *Lowered risk of neurodegenerative diseases*

- *Extended lifespan*

- *Decreased blood pressure and cholesterol readings*

---

[227] http://pepbk.co/TheMBTD

- *Reduced of insulin resistance*

- *Faster metabolism*

A little-known secret taught in both of my books (*The Metabolic Blowtorch Diet* and **Guaranteed Shredded**[228]) is melting stubborn body fat via catecholamine activation from 18–24-hour fast intervals.

This increases the adrenal gland's production of the fight or flight hormones: epinephrine, norepinephrine, noradrenaline and adrenaline.

Afterwards, this triggers a cascade of physiological responses, including an increase in temperature, heart rate, respiration rate and energy expenditure which over time leads to a decrease in stored body fat.

Here's the simple explanation of why this is important[229]:

> *"To burn, or "mobilize," stored body fat, your body produces chemicals known as **catecholamines** (also known as fight or flight hormones).*
>
> *These molecules travel through your blood and "attach" to receptors on fat cells, which trigger the release of heat stored within the cells to be*

[228] http://pepbk.co/GuaranteedShredded
[229] http://pepbk.co/StubbornFat

burned for energy.

Fat cells have two types of receptors for catecholamines: alpha- and beta-receptors.

To keep this simple, beta-receptors speed up fat mobilization, whereas alpha- receptors hinder it.

And here's the big difference between "regular" and "stubborn" fat:

Fat that is easy to lose has more beta-receptors than alpha.

Fat that is hard to lose has more alpha-receptors than beta.*"*

Stubborn body fat doesn't come off unless your body is in fight or flight response mode.

When one fasts for 18-24 hours or longer, the body attacks (via the activation of catecholamines) the stubborn body fat deposits and reduces them over time."

By adding "low impact, steady state cardio"[230] in the beginning and end of these fast windows (intervals) your results are effectively doubly potent for incinerating stubborn fat stores.

---

[230] http://pepbk.co/TOTAndCardio

For a comprehensive explanation of this process, read my best-selling book on the topic, **The Metabolic Blowtorch Diet**[231].

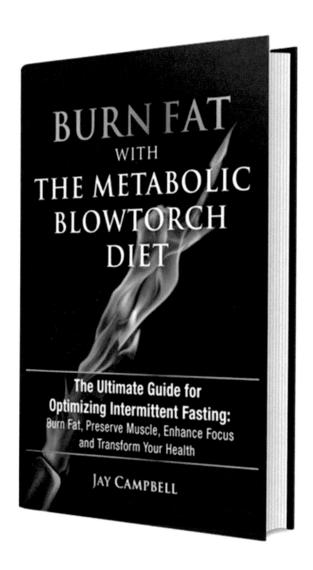

[231] http://pepbk.co/TheMBTD

Thank you so much for finishing this book and reading to the end.

I hope you found this information valuable and will put it to use ASAP.

It is my sincere desire you can become a meta human with the ability to look like this:

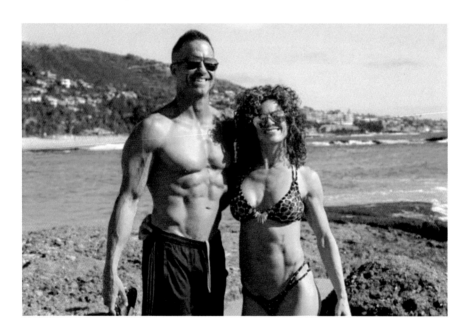

RESOURCES PAGE

My Website[232]

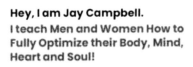 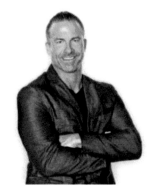

Jump into the Jay Campbell ecosystem and allow me to help you optimize your body, mind, heart and soul.

---

[232] http://pepbk.co/JayCampbell

Fully Optimized Health[233]

Join my private membership group and gain state-of-the-art testosterone optimization, cutting-edge intel on peptides, fat loss, muscle building, gray market agents while also learning how to raise your vibration.

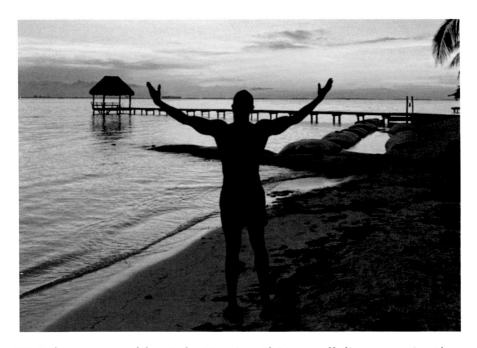

Watch my weekly Ask Me Anything call live or via the recordings.

---

[233] http://pepbk.co/FullyOptimizedHealth

The Top 10 Questions To Ask Your Doctor About Therapeutic Testosterone[234] (Free)

Know all the red flags to watch out for *before* your appointment by keeping yourself informed of the top 10 questions to ask your doctor.

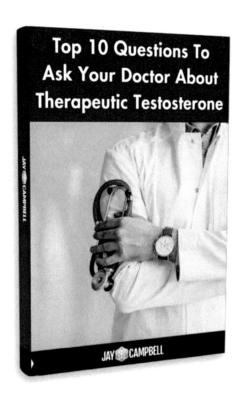

---

[234] http://pepbk.co/TOTD-10Mistakes

The Top 10 Mistakes People Make When Starting Peptides[235] (Free)

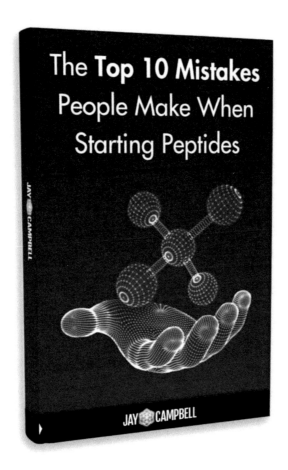

Avoid the trial and error experienced by 95% of peptide users and learn how to supercharge your results.

---

[235] http://pepbk.co/ThePeptidesCourse-10Mistakes

Consult with me[236]

Speak with me to overcome a serious issue or to further tweak and enhance your current protocol.

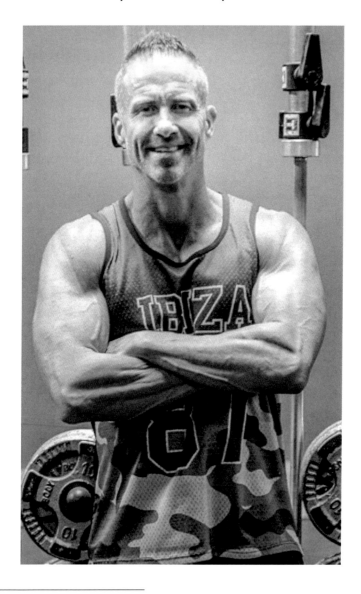

[236] http://pepbk.co/ConsultWithMe

Hire me as your personal, 1-on-1 optimization coach[237]

From time to time, I allow people to join my VIP Insider Circle where I dive DEEP to help you become the highest and best version of yourself.

Fill out the application form to see you're qualified to work with Jay as a VIP Mastermind client.

---

[237] http://pepbk.co/VIP

Train exactly like I do by training to Positive Muscle Failure[238]

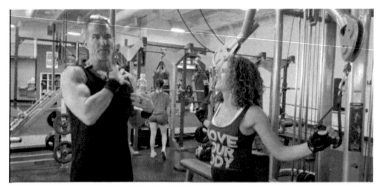

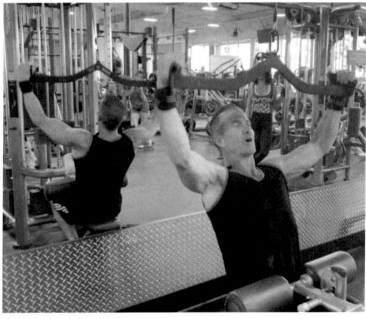

Learn how to tax all three energy systems to build maximum muscle in minimum time with my video workout programs.

---

[238] http://pepbk.co/PMFTraining

Check out my product recommendations[239]

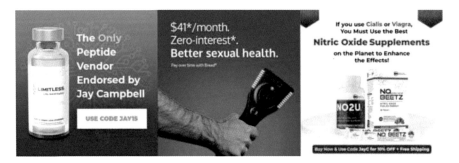

Learn the exact peptides, supplements, and tools I use to help people become fully optimized.

Save up to 15% by using the affiliate codes listed.

---

[239] http://pepbk.co/Recommendations

TO CONNECT WITH JAY ONLINE:

Website: **pepbk.co/JayCampbell**

Youtube: **pepbk.co/YouTube**

Newsletter: **pepbk.co/Newsletter**

Twitter: **pepbk.co/Twitter**

Instagram: **pepbk.co/Instagram**

TikTok: **pepbk.co/TikTok**

LinkedIn: **pepbk.co/LinkedIn**

Made in United States
Orlando, FL
01 August 2024

49694274R00148